# CONTENTS

# YOU ARE BEAUTIFUL

## A New Perspective on Health and Nutrition

Philip Bryden

Mush Nutrition

## Mush Nutrition Publications

This book contains advice and information relating to health care. It is not intended to replace medical advice and should be used to supplement rather than replace regular care by your doctor. It is recommended that you seek your physician's advice before embarking on any medical program or treatment. You are advised to consult with your health care professional with regard to matters relating to your health, and in particular regarding matters that may require diagnosis or medical attention. The author disclaims any liability for any medical outcome that may occur as a result of applying the methods suggested in this book.

Mush Nutrition
www.mushnutrition.com
Cover photo by Philip Bryden

*Dedicated to the memory of James and Janice Bryden.*

*The Beginning*

F ood is an essential component in my childhood memories. From the greasy hamburgers
that my father and I would order on the beach
in Santa Monica to the bowls of popcorn that my
mother would make as we settled in to watch TV
as a family on Saturday night, my childhood was
filled with food. Family vacations were always punc-
tuated with favourite restaurants, bakeries, and ice
cream shops. Food was for pleasure and taste gratification. Healthy nutrition was almost a happy coincidence. The preventable illnesses that precipitated
my father's death were all related to his food choices.

The following is a glimpse into personal recollec-
tions, nutritional awareness, and some basic concepts of Eastern thought. By seeing ourselves as holistic beings, we can better understand our health and
more effectively influence the course of our lives. We
are not reductive parts of a whole. We are the whole.
Optimal health is not an accident, but rather stems
from conscious decisions. Longevity and disease can
surely be affected by genetics, yet we can greatly
influence the path of individual health. Traditional

Philip Bryden

Western medicine widely treats nutrition as an afterthought in the prevention, recognition, and diagnosis of disease. Nutrition, however, is key. It is the fuel that runs our factories. The influence of nutrition over all aspects of our personal lives is vast. Every morsel of food that we consume affects our bodies and our minds. Personal wellbeing is a choice, which begins with the food that we put in to our bodies.

## CHAPTER ONE

*A Brief History, Part I*

**M**y father died in March 2014 as the direct result of a multitude of self-inflicted, preventable diseases. He drove casually past the first warning light of his eventual physical demise in 1991, when he suffered a heart attack at the age of 61. He spent a few days in the hospital that year to undergo routine surgery to place stents in his arteries. These would keep his arteries open and functioning properly. The cardiologist prescribed medication and recommended reducing stress levels, advising him to take up some form of low impact exercise. My father's eating habits were never discussed or questioned.

After his heart attack, my father left his job and worked as a part-time consultant for the next few years, until being ungraciously moved aside by the industry in which he had spent most of his professional life. Working for a subsidiary of NASA, he was involved in the first launches of satellites and precursors to the Apollo space missions. My father was involved in the MJS project, the first fly-by reconnaissance of Mars, Jupiter, and Saturn. When funding for NASA hit the skids during the first few years of the first Reagan Administration, he moved with great reticence from the liberal, scientific world of space exploration to the ultra-conservative, military world of defence contracting. Rather than interacting with other engineers and scientists who looked to the skies for their inspiration, he was now in meetings with government and military officials to develop armament tools during the final years of the Cold War. This was a difficult transition for a lifelong defender of liberal politics. An increased travel schedule went hand in hand with an increased level of internal conflict. He was essentially working for the other side, and he did not enjoy it. My father always accepted irony in life as foundational, but this was difficult for him to tolerate. He stuck with it as best he could. This was 1982, nine years prior to his heart attack.

Stress and conflicted emotions were not the only contributors to that first yellow warning light. My father had a dangerous relationship with food. He ate for pleasure. Much like an alcoholic sneaking drinks from hidden bottles around the house, he snuck foods – unhealthy foods. My father sought compensation and comfort through addictive foods. These would include processed meats (lots of processed meats), difficult to find exotic cheeses (he would claim that these reminded him of his childhood growing up in Europe), along with bread, elaborate pastries and ice creams (special treats that seemed to be special on a very regular basis). His guilty pleasures were the delicatessens and the pastry shops. My father smoked when he was a younger man, but quit before he was forty. He rarely drank alcohol. My father's burden was what he put on his plate, and subsequently into his body on a recurring and excessive basis. Once a svelte man in his thirties, he regularly carried an excess of twenty to sixty pounds after he turned forty.

My father would undergo a second operation to replace the stents that had been put in after his first heart attack. This measure was normal preventative medical maintenance to replace aging parts before they could wear out on their own. The stents and daily heart medication kept the problems at bay allowing him to enjoy his somewhat precipitated retirement and the first pair of his young grandchildren. He did, however, continue to carry excessive weight. The NutriSystem and Weight Watcher food replacement diets that the doctors recommended were frustrating and ineffective. His frustration led to an increased craving for the same, unhealthy foods, which cascaded into more binge eating and clandestine snacking. The spinning wheel of disease was well in place and was picking up speed at a dizzying rate. My father's eating habits were never discussed or questioned.

Over the next decade, my father would be treated for high blood pressure, diagnosed with Type-2 diabetes and would have his gall bladder removed. Just a reminder, the gall bladder controls the release of bile, which is responsible for the breaking down of fats as they head in to the small intestine. His new ailments required new medicines, some of which were prescribed only to offset the negative side effects of the new drugs themselves. An entire shelf in the kitchen cabinet was dedicated to his pill containers. Many of the pills, all covered by Medicare and Medicaid, looked alike and my father was easily confused. He was getting older and the doctors reassured him that his confusion was normal. My father's eating habits were never discussed or questioned.

In 2010, my father began to experience a new repertory of symptoms – blood in his stool, difficult digestion, nausea, and abdominal pain. He underwent a colonoscopy, which revealed some polyps in his lower intestine. These were diagnosed as pre-cancerous and removed. More medications were prescribed. New growths were discovered over time and treated locally. Thus, began a cascade of grave digestive issues that ultimately led to an attempt at chemotherapy treatment, and resulted in a major surgical intervention.

My father had been diagnosed with cancer of the colon. Both of his parents had died from the disease; his father at the age of 49, and his mother in her mid-70s. My father had always viewed this affliction as an inevitable dark cloud in his life. The doctors had referred to colon cancer as an inherited disease, only somewhat unavoidable, and had never considered lifestyle as being a contributing factor. My father's eating habits were never discussed or questioned.

As defined by the National Institute of Diabetes and Digestive and Kidney Disorders (NIDDK), "Ostomy surgery of the bowel, also known as bowel diversion, refers to surgical procedures that reroute the normal movement of intestinal contents out of the body when part of the bowel is diseased or removed. Creating an ostomy means bringing part of the intestine through the abdominal wall so that waste exits through the abdominal wall instead of passing through the anus."

*Colostomy* (lower colon) or *ileostomy* (entire lower gastro-intestinal tract) surgery can be temporary or permanent, depending upon the gravity of the situation. An ileostomy is when the surgeon removes or bypasses the entire colon, rectum, and anus. My father underwent a permanent ileostomy. The final eight months of my father's medically prolonged life were confused and painful. He lived in a permanent no man's land between compromised human dignity and unrelenting survival instincts that left him emotionally and mentally paralysed.

My father's reliance and unwavering belief in the absolute power of the "white coats" of the medical profession prevented him from attempting any other treatments. In his final months, my father would have to receive bi-weekly intravenous hydration. Along with its job of waste removal, the lower GI tract is also the primary site for micronutrient (vitamins and minerals) and water absorption, both crucial to human survival. My father no longer possessed this body part. His oncologist suggested that he simply drink sufficient liquids to thwart dehydration issues. He even confirmed that any liquid would do the job, and went on to list the following: coffee, tea, fruit juices, sodas, and only lastly, water. When none of these liquids worked to sufficiently hydrate him, routine of IV hydration began.

Thus was the undignified end to my father's life. His relationship with food, his dismissal of nutritional influence on his health, and his absolute reliance on the medical establishment all combined to create the slow and steady destruction of his body. My father's accumulated diseases were preventable. The plethora of warning lights that flashed during his last twenty years were medically treated one by one, but no substantial changes were ever made to his lifestyle. My father finally succumbed to the relentless slow burn of disease on April 15th, confirming the old adage, "Nothing is ever certain but death and taxes." He would have appreciated the irony.

As I meandered my way through undergraduate studies at UCLA, I became increasingly preoccupied with personal health and individual sports. I rode my bicycle as if I were training for competitive races even though this was not always the case. I kept a mileage and timing journal of my rides. I also kept a food diary. I would record what I ate, how much I ate, when I ate, and, to some extent, even why I ate! I enjoyed the discipline and obscurity of those habits. Eventually, I began to follow a strict plant-based diet. Just because...

After graduating with a degree in Cinema in the mid-eighties, I started bicycle touring in Europe, and ultimately worked as a guide for long distance cyclotourism rides, even traveling to many of the then re-emerging Eastern Block countries. I had grown up hearing my grandparents and family friends speaking with different European accents. English was the second language to nearly all of that generation of my relatives. It was no surprise that I felt more of an affinity for life in Europe than I did for life in Los Angeles, despite having been born and raised there. The world was a large place, and I wanted to see as much of it as possible. I think that, subconsciously, I also wanted to break patterns, and I knew that I would have to get myself out of the fish bowl before I could try to swim in the ocean.

I moved to France in the early nineties and based myself there. At that time, French food culture was heavily resistant to vegetarianism. People would react with shock when I would tell them that I didn't eat meat, fish, eggs, or cheese. Mon Dieu! No cheese? This is France...! It felt like I was almost an insult to the integrity of the nation. Overall, there were far fewer available animal-free choices than what I had known in California (this is luckily no longer the case). I also had less nutritional knowledge back then. I struggled to maintain my somewhat random, plant-based diet, and, after putting up a short-lived resistance, I reluctantly went back to eating meat, fish, eggs, and, yes, even cheese.

I began working in television, and quickly specialised in covering live sports events, from horse racing to tennis to the Tour de France. Over the years, I witnessed and documented various epic sporting events. Sometimes I had the best seat in the house, and oftentimes on the field of play in direct contact with some of the world's elite athletes. I was there to witness the drug-aided victories of Lance Armstrong. I saw spectacular rides from the world's elite jockeys, and I documented stunning triumphs from tennis players like Roger Federer and Serena Williams, amongst others. The obscurity of my college journaling habits seemed to make sense in this world where discipline and sacrifice for the sake of physical achievement were considered normal.

◆ ◆ ◆

My father was born in Switzerland in 1930. His name was Tobias. His father, Eugen, was a German stage director. His mother, Sonja, was a Jewish actress from Romania. Eugen worked with the Vienna and Salzburg opera companies. He was the stage director for numerous productions and international tours. Eugen was a prolific artist. Sonja was a celebrated stage actress. She spoke Romanian and German. The marriage between a high-profile German director and a celebrated Jewish actress, however, was a risky proposition, given the extreme political tensions brewing in Europe at the time. Eugen and Sonja were clever, however, and decided to go to Bern, Switzerland for the birth of their son, my father. They wanted to have a Swiss passport in the family. This was their insurance policy in case of political emergency.

As a family, they lived in Vienna, Austria. Eugen and Sonja worked there, and my father went to school there. In 1937, anti-Semitism was rife and extreme right politics were experiencing a strong and prolonged groundswell. Eugen was on tour with an opera in the United States. He knew that this was the perfect and perhaps only opportunity to get his family out of Europe safely. He was already out, and that was the most difficult part of the equation. He sent a cryptic, but clearly understandable telegram to his wife in Vienna. It was time to leave. As they were not an anonymous family, Sonja and Tobias would have to depart with only a small suitcase as if they were heading off for a weekend trip. They would close the door on their home and belongings in Vienna. They would never return.

The Swiss passport turned out to be invaluable. With the help of Eugen's tenuous political connections and a trustworthy uncle, Sonja and Tobias were able to get through to the Swiss border, cross Switzerland into France, and get across France to the seaport of La Rochelle. They were to meet Eugen in Cuba, where they would await approval of their immigration visas into the United States. This process would take two years.

Eugen had become close friends with a couple of New York actors. They would prove to be instrumental in the immigration process, providing letters of recommendation and offering logistical solutions as the need arose. They remained close family friends for the years to come.

During the Cuba interim, Eugen painted incessantly. He observed and recorded the people, the streets, and the moments of Cuban life that surrounded him. Everything was new and very different from the European artistic world he had known from his previous life. He was inspired. He was free. Eugen, Sonja, and Tobias learned Spanish together. This was their new life, at least for the moment, and they found themselves in a constant state of flux. New languages, new places, new opportunities. There was nothing around them to remind them of their past. It was an uncertain time period; sometimes disturbing. It was also exhilarating. Tobias spent every day with his parents. He was a young boy in a new place. His eyes were wide open. He forged a close bond with his father, who, from all accounts, was an exuberant, talented, and playful man. Tobias enjoyed these years in Cuba, as would any child. His parents were free from work constraints and his school hours were limited to say the least. They were the outsiders and they enjoyed this status.

Once their immigration visas were approved, they headed to the States. Eugen and Sonja were not yet forty, and, for all intents and purposes, had the best of their careers ahead of them. Eugen knew two people in New York. Sonja and Tobias arrived into a land of complete strangers. This is when things would change drastically. Germany was in the throes of Hitler's deadly rise to power. It was not necessarily a good thing to be a German in the United States. Eugen, Sonja, and Tobias had a strong desire to fit in to the society of this new country that had opened its doors to them. They were all getting new American passports. Their old passports would be cut in half and thrown away. This was the time to create a new identity if ever there was such a time. Eugen changed his family name from the very German sounding Schulz to Breiden (the maiden name of his first wife), which eventually became Americanized to Bryden. Tobias was told that he could choose a new given name as well. They wanted to erase all outward signs of their European past. My father chose the name James. Tobias was gone.

Over the next few years, the transition to life in the United States would prove to be a complicated one. Eugen and Sonja had gone from being celebrated, somewhat public figures in the European cultural mecca of Vienna, to being unknowns in Manhattan, a city overrun with stage directors and actresses looking for work. Nothing was moving forward for either of them on a professional level. They decided that, to increase their chances of success, it would be judicious for Eugen to head to Los Angeles to seek work while Sonja and James would stay in New York. Despite letters of recommendation and glowing references from some of the entertainment industry's most visible figures, nothing really changed for either Eugen or Sonja. To make ends meet, Sonja would eventually work as a housekeeper in Manhattan. In

Los Angeles, Eugen persisted in his pursuit of a job worthy of his talent and experience. He was proud and stubborn, with high standards. After a year, the family finally reunited in Los Angeles. Eugen would direct one stage play. Sonja would be cast in one film, directed by an old friend from Europe, Max Ophuls. James would change schools seventeen times before graduating from high school.

Shortly after James's high school graduation, Eugen died from cancer at the age of 49. James was devastated. He quickly realised that he was now responsible not only for his own life, but for that of his mother, a fifty year-old unemployed actress with a heavy German accent. James had to step up. The Korean War was gathering speed, and James decided that he would rather enlist in the Air Force than be drafted into the Army. The Air Force, he figured, would give him more skills with which to get work after his service. James also felt a great deal of gratitude toward the United States; the country that had given he and his parents a fresh start. This is a feeling that he would carry with him throughout his life. He spent his required time in the service before starting college, where he pursued a double major in math and physics. James obtained his Bachelor's Degree from UCLA in three years.

Rather than pursuing his passions, James had become obsessed with stability. From the moment his father died, he dedicated his life to overcoming the disjointed and disrupted childhood that he had experienced. James was adored by his parents and had been a happy, although solitary child. He also saw first-hand the difficulties that came along with pursuing one's dreams. His father had been proud and obstinate in his career, and life had been more difficult because of it. His mother had gone from being a celebrated actress to doing odd jobs for other people. James vowed that he wanted something different. He pursued a profession that offered stability, and dedicated a vast amount of energy to creating a comfortable, stable home for his family. He was present as a father, and reliable as a husband. James remained a caring and responsible son, and Sonja was a stirring presence in our family life until she passed. James had few friends. He never spoke of his father.

My father saw life as something that happens to you. You do your best to roll with the punches. Life is a pinball game, and you're the pinball. This had been his experience. Survive. Keep expectations realistic. Do not dream. My father's view of human existence was a fatalistic one. He did not feel that you could meaningfully influence anything that might happen to you. You try to manage the cards that you have been dealt. If it's a great hand, play it quickly. If the cards are bad, bluff. And if you're going to bluff, the only way is to go all in. This is how he viewed his own life, and this is how he treated his health.

Much as my father's adult choices were in opposition to the lives of his parents, and my path would also be in direct contrast to how my own parents lived. Every child must decide whether to walk in accordance with his or her upbringing, or you walk in the opposite direction. I decided to take chances. I decided to turn away from stability, to make decisions that did not always put me on the path of least resistance, and sometimes these choices were to my own detriment. I chose to try things that were difficult, and to play my own hand with the cards I had been given. No bluffing. No over-betting. No excuses. I chose to take control over the things that I *could* control. What I would create, what I would put into the world, what I would put into my consciousness, and what I would put into my body. The latter, I found, would dictate everything else.

## CHAPTER TWO

*The Whole Person*

*The Cambridge Dictionary* defines *holistic* as *"relating to the whole of something or to the total system instead of just to its parts. Holistic medicine attempts to treat the whole person, including the mind and body, not just the injury or disease."*

## HOLISTIC MEDECINE – THE QUEST FOR BALANCE

Western medicine is a system built around finding a cure. You go to the doctor, you describe your symptoms, the doctor gives you a prescription to treat the symptoms, and those symptoms eventually or hopefully disappear. If they do not disappear, then you return to the doctor and alternate medications can be prescribed in an attempt to alleviate the symptoms. Western medicine treats the symptom of an ailment, but rarely the cause of the ailment.

There are doctors for every specific part and function of the body, all expertly trained, and highly specialised. There are cardiologists, dermatologists, endocrinologists, gastroenterologists, nephrologists, neurologists, oncologists, ophthalmologists, pulmonologists, rheumatologists, and urologists, just to name a few. These medical doctors are all necessary for the specific research and treatment of their specific and individual branches of medicine. If your physician is not able to offer a solution to the symptom, it is highly likely that he or she will refer you to a specialist, and that specialist will look more deeply into his or her field of expertise to solve the symptom, or possibly refer you to an even more specialised specialist. This seems like an efficient system, a sort of sifting of the sand of human ailments - the finer the grains, the smaller the sifter, and so on. This telescopic approach to human health and conventional medical research generally looks at the components rather than recognising and examining their interconnections. The parts receive greater attention than the whole.

Holistic medicine is a form of healing that considers the whole person – body, mind, spirit, and emotions – in the quest for optimal health. Ideally, each individual strives for optimal health by gaining balance in the physical body and in everyday life. The human body can be viewed as a complex factory; if one part is not working properly, all the other parts will be affected.

Imbalances in the individual can affect overall health and the causes of these imbalances must be identified. Of course, medications can be effective to relieve aggravated symptoms, but a holistic approach to cure and prevent further problems would require an eventual lifestyle change. These changes can and usually do necessitate new nutritional choices. What goes into the factory will have a direct impact on how efficiently the factory operates.

In the United States, medical education generally consists of at least three years of *pre-med* courses. Pre-med is followed by four years of *second entry degrees*, at the conclusion of which, a degree of Doctor of Medicine (M.D.) is granted. Over those seven years of study to become a practicing medical doctor, an average of less than 25 hours of study is dedicated to nutrition.

In a 2004 survey on nutritional education in medical schools, all 126 accredited medical schools in the United States were queried. According to *The American Journal of Clinical Nutrition*, which conducted the survey, "*a total of 106 surveys were returned. Ninety-nine of the 106 schools responding required some form of nutrition education; however, only 32 schools (30%) required a separate nutrition course. On average, students received 23.9 contact hours of nutrition during medical school (range 2-70 hours). Only 40 schools required the minimum 25 hours recommended by the National Academy of Sciences.*" Nearly 90% of all professors in these medical schools admitted that nutrition should be given more attention in the curriculum. This survey goes on to state "...the bulk of nutrition education continues to be taught in the basic science course or in an integrated format. This means that three-quarters of the nutrition instruction in medical schools is not specifically identified as nutrition in the curriculum." *(from "Status of nutrition education in medical schools" Kelly M Adams, Karen C Lindell, and Steven H Zeisel).*

There is an immense amount of education and instruction on how the components of the factory work; however, there is virtually no information about what raw materials ensure the proper functioning of these components or their whole. Details receive preference over the big picture. The leaf gets preference not only over the tree, but also over the entire forest. It is like looking through a telescope to identify the person sitting next to you.

The impact of nutrition on human health is desperately neglected by most medical professionals, as proven by the feeble amount of time that doctors receive in medical education. Yet, health starts with food. Food can either promote disease or prevent disease. Ask your physician about preventing and curing ailments with food. You will most likely be met with some form of dismissal. This reaction may simply be due to lack of knowledge. After all, 23 hours over a seven-year education doesn't weigh in very heavily. Also, there is no real benefit to the doctor if patients are able to prevent illnesses. Doctors would soon be out of business. There is no real reason for the pharmaceutical industry to promote holistic or alternative approaches to health and disease prevention. Those companies would soon be out of business.

The only one who has anything to gain is the patient, and what business owner would willingly empower his customers so that they would never return to his business?

A holistic perspective of personal health is as necessary as it is difficult to come by in Western countries and cultures. It can be as simple as taking the proverbial step back. Look at the whole picture, the whole person. It is impossible to separate the healthy functioning of the body's systems from one another, and it is perilous to isolate symptoms of illnesses without addressing their causes. If the goal of medical professionals is to work toward attaining and maintaining optimal health for each individual, then it is only logical that a comprehensive view of the individual should be primordial to the medical profession. A holistic approach to health helps to empower each person to understand and influence the root causes of many discomforts and diseases. It helps him or her to comprehend the idea that personal actions and choices are as great a contributor to disease as are bacteria and viruses.

## DIVERSITY – APPRECIATING DIFFERENCES

Diversity is perhaps one of the finest words that can be used for the human race. We are all members of the same species with the same physical components. The size, shape, and colour of these components may change, but these are mere details. Our bodies all work in the same way. The different factories are built with nearly identical parts. We all have and need lungs for breathing, a heart to control blood flow and circulation, a brain to oversee proper body function and handle emotional integration, skin (regardless of its colour) to help wrap the whole package and to help control body temperature. We all have the same set of muscles, and our skeletons all have 207 bones. The bottom line is that all humans possess the same organs, and that these organs are responsible for the same functions in each individual being. As a species, we are fairly homogenous on a purely functional level. Most of our factories operate smoothly and without struggle; some, though, may experience punctual or permanent challenges on a physical or emotional level.

Within all of this relative physical sameness, however, reside numerous differences that are highly individual and constantly susceptible to experiencing changes. Culture, language, family, religion, gender, and education, are among the numerous external environmental characteristics that differentiate one human being from another. Each individual also possesses his or her unique set of physical characteristics that help to differentiate him or her from other people. These specific traits involve the shape and colour of the eyes, the thickness and colour of the hair, height, weight, skin colour, the size and shape of the nose, the timbre of the voice, amongst millions of other highly individual characteristics. Each person has a different body type. Specifics of body type combined with unique environmental conditions and characteristics mix together in each person to create an amazingly diverse species.

A holistic view of a person involves all of these characteristics. Conventional medicine would strive to unify the differences, to analyse the parts rather than the whole. A malfunctioning liver, for example, might be treated with prescribed medication or surgical intervention in the same way for a sedentary urban European, an Alaskan Inuit, a professional athlete, or a nomadic Saharan Tuareg. After all, a liver is a liver. This isolationist view of a faltering body part may be clinically accurate. The problem might be solved, but the cause might remain untreated, thus opening the door to a recurrence of the initial malfunction or even the breakdown of a different body part or function that receives the wrath of the still untreated cause. A holistic diagnosis for the cure and the prevention of further disease of the malfunctioning liver would certainly analyse the problematic organ, but would also incorporate environmental conditions, emotional and mental states, as well as body type to fully understand and treat the ailment. This approach would allow for the implementation of long-term positive actions. It would help the individual to understand the various physical phenomena that arise in his or her body over time, and it would empower personal change as a means of prevention and treatment.


## AYURVEDA – BALANCE AND THE DOSHAS

The Oxford English Dictionary defines Ayurveda as *"The traditional Hindu system of medicine (incorporated in Atharva Veda, the last of the four Vedas), which is based on the idea of balance in bodily systems and uses diet, herbal treatment, and yogic breathing."* Merriam-Webster defines Ayurveda as *"a form of alternative medicine that is the traditional system of medicine of India and seeks to treat and integrate body, mind, and spirit using a holistic approach especially by emphasizing diet, herbal remedies, exercise, meditation, breathing, and physical therapy."* The origins of Ayurveda have been traced to 6,000 BCE as an oral tradition and approximately 2,000 BCE in a written form. Ayurveda is still widely practiced today (it is integrated as part of the Indian National health care system), and is thus the oldest existing health care system in the world. In traditional Sanskrit language, *ãyurevedah*, from *ãyuh* life + *vedah* knowledge. Life Knowledge.

Body type is a key element in the practice of Ayurveda. Each individual is born with a predominant body type, or *dosha*, which includes all of the physical aspects of the individual. There are three doshas: *Vita, Pitta,* and *Kapha.* Each person possesses qualities from all three doshas, with physical characteristics as a foundational criterion to establish the predominant dosha. Environmental characteristics (family situation, work environment, relationships, diet...) also contribute to the composition of a person's dosha. As one's predominant physical dosha inevitably encounters environmental factors, the dominance of one dosha over the other two will be variable over time. Change is inevitable and continuous as environmental factors are rarely constant. The goal is to strive for balance between the doshas. One cannot control all, or any, environmental factors; one can only control the manner in which he attempts to deal with them. Balance is a principle factor in the pursuit of optimal health. It is thus fundamental to consider all components of an individual while working toward this objective.

A person cannot consciously determine the genetic, physical characteristics that he receives at birth. Implants, facelifts, plastic surgeries, and hair dyes are merely costumes. Although some of these are more permanent then others, they do not truly change inherent traits. Environmental influences are primarily out of our control, lest the ways in which we receive and perceive them. So, how do we enact change in order to offer greater balance to factors seemingly or realistically beyond our reach? There is one outside factor well within our realm of choice and control that affects both the physical being and the environmental factors with which we live. The food that we choose to consume has far reaching consequences for our physical and mental health, our perceptions of self and others, and our pursuit of the grail of personal balance. Disease prevention and cure, physical performance, and emotional and mental wellbeing can all be hugely influenced by the foods that we choose to put into our bodies.

## FOOD IS MEDICINE

Hippocrates, the Greek physician, who lived over 2,000 years ago, famously stated, *"Let thy food be thy medicine, and thy medicine be thy food."* This is the same Hippocrates to whom all graduating Western medical doctors must pledge the sacred oath of their profession to uphold fundamental ethical standards. A fundamental premise of Ayurvedic philosophy is that *"food is medicine and medicine is food."* Both of these ancient principles with regard to food and personal health are identical. Another Ayurvedic proverb states that *"when diet is wrong, medicine is of no use; when diet is correct, medicine is of no need."* It all comes back to food. 24.9 hours of nutritional education over the course of seven-years of medical school in order to become a doctor. This seems a paltry allotment of time for such a crucial element of overall health. While the continuing advances in modern medicine are undeniable, remarkable, and progressive in terms of the diagnosis and treatment of disease, these same advances tend to disarm and distance the individual from his own state of health. What an individual puts into his body can determine his state of being - physically, mentally, and emotionally. Nutrition is the foundation for the empowerment to influence personal health.


## PREVENTION OVER CURE

The reason that people take medicine is because there is some sort of malfunction, weakness, disease, or pain in the body. Identifying the location of the ailment, pinpointing the affected organ or body system, selecting the desired treatment, anticipating eventual complications, crossing fingers. Medicine, whether it's conventional, Chinese, or Ayurveda, involves a certain level of trial and error that is inherent to attempting to cure an ailment. No doctor holds magic powers. He can neither read the future nor see the past. He suggests solutions with possible or even probable outcomes, based upon past experience and research. Usually, when a person goes to see a doctor or a specialist, it is because there is already a problem that needs to be resolved. The next step is a sort of race against time to try to eradicate the problem as quickly as possible. Few people go to the doctor when they are feeling well. The doctor has a role similar to that of a bomb squad for the body. There is a ticking clock wired to five sticks of dynamite that needs to be disarmed before it explodes.

What if there was no time bomb? What if there was a greatly reduced need to take medications and drugs to solve physical and mental problems? What if the answer to public and individual health problems lay in easily implemented changes and basic education? What if the foods we eat could prevent and cure disease? What if each individual was able to prolong his life and greatly diminish the risk of preventable diseases? These questions may sound idyllic and naïve, but there are easy-to-implement measures that could lead to positive responses for all of them. These answers lie in the foods we eat, when we eat them, and how we eat them.

Whole plant foods contain a vast array of naturally occurring medicinal compounds that can positively affect personal health. The human body did not evolve with a reliance on synthetic medications as part of the master plan. Nor did it evolve due to the benefits of refined and processed foods. It did not evolve based upon the availability of packaged foods with extended shelf lives. High fructose corn syrup, nitrate preservatives, artificial flavourings and colourings are not part of our genetic nutritional needs. The consumption of animal flesh and dairy products is for taste, not health. In our quest for convenience and foods that satisfy the unhealthy cravings that they actually help to perpetuate, modern society has neglected health for instant gratification with no consideration for the inevitable negative consequences that these choices hold. The foods that we choose to consume either prevent or promote disease. Salt, sugar, and saturated fat create addictive responses, especially when combined and fried, and increase the risk of chronic heart disease, obesity, insulin resistance, and chronic inflammation. These are examples of disease promoters. Whole grains, organic fruits and vegetables, and nuts and seeds contain dietary fibre, vitamins and minerals, healthy fats and carbohydrates, as well as high concentrations of antioxidants that help to reduce the frequency and likelihood of chronic ailments. These are examples of disease preventers. Food can act as preventative and curative medicine. Of course, it would be reductive to claim that food alone is the health solution to every ailment, illness, or disease. It is possible, however, to stack the deck in your favour by eating foods that promote health rather than destroy it.

## *LIFE KNOWLEDGE*

Life Knowledge. The more knowledge one has about something, the better equipped he is to understand it and have the possibility to make the best choices. These favourable decisions are not always made, however, despite the knowledge. This is free will. Life knowledge does not mean fortune telling or crystal balls informing a person of what is going to happen in life, nor is it an empirical set of rules that dictate behaviour. Life knowledge is about trying to understand how everything works, and, more specifically, how everything works for the individual. This is not finite knowledge, and should be understood as truly infinite, meaning that there is never a point at which complete understanding has been achieved. This would be impossible, as the parameters for this knowledge are constantly evolving. The more things that we strive to understand about ourselves, the better equipped we are to avoid and solve problems, make positive, proactive decisions, and lead slightly more empowered lives.

## *ADAPTATION - KNOWLEDGE IS POWER*

As human beings, we are not just a bag of parts. Each person is a unique blend of physical, psychological, emotional, mental, and environmental factors. The continuous quest for understanding as to how all of these elements fit together, and the comprehension that events in our lives are somehow based upon the ebb and flow of numerous individual factors allows for a clearer vision as to how we can influence what happens to us. Think of an experienced surfer going into the ocean. First, he looks at the water, checks the wind, and acknowledges the temperature. He assesses the conditions. This is the first point of influence from which he will make his next decisions. These elements are out of his control, yet within his realm of understanding, and they will help him to determine his next move. Wetsuit or no wetsuit. Long board or short board. These are decisions for which the individual is entirely responsible. He is making choices based upon information, knowledge, previous experience, and personal choice. Once he is in the water, all of the previous decisions and calculations serve as his tools. Sets of waves will come and go, the water current may change, and the wind may shift. Again, these parameters are entirely out of his control. He must now determine how he reacts to these elements. He decides which wave to ride, where to sit in the water to be in the ideal spot for the next set. He constantly adapts and adjusts his actions and decisions to fit his conditions as is best for him at that precise moment. What was once the best place might gradually or suddenly deteriorate, and he will alter his perspective, reassess, and reposition accordingly. All of these choices might be entirely different for another surfer, even one who comes to surf in the same waters.

## *AYURVEDA – LIFE KNOWLEDGE*

The vocation of Ayurveda, Life Knowledge, is "alleviating both bodily and mental diseases and promoting both physical and psychological well-being." *(Yoga and Ayurveda, David Frawley).* The nutritional foundation of Ayurveda is based on the idea that you are the result of what, when, where, how, and why you eat. Ayurveda explains that food should be eaten mindfully and with gratitude, and that it should be fresh, of the highest quality, digestible, delicious, lovingly prepared, and satisfying to your senses. Ayurveda offers a balanced approach to preparing, eating, and digesting your food based on your unique dosha, as well as the time of day, the season, your life cycle, and where you live. Ayurvedic nutrition is truly holistic nutrition. The dietary practices that lie within also encourage a conscious way of living. This applies to food and to life in a larger sense as well. Ayurveda is a way of embracing food as life-giving energy. It is a way of understanding how your individual nature and the unique set of influences around you help to determine how well your food choices will serve you. Ayurveda explains that your dietary needs and your subsequent digestion of nutrients are affected by the rhythms of nature, your individual constitution, and the changes that occur in your life. The surfer and his wave.

## *PRANA - LIFE FORCE*

*Prana* is the Sanskrit word meaning "life force." In Ayurveda, prana refers to the organic energy that permeates reality on all levels. Merriam-Webster defines prana as "a life breath in Vedic and later Hindu religion; the principle of life moving in the human body." In living beings, this universal energy is thought to be responsible for all bodily functions through five different types of prana. These are collectively known as the *vayus,* or the paths of vital circulation that exist throughout the body.

Prana can also be thought of as breath. The process

of inhaling and exhaling is essential, and is the only crossover bodily function that can be controlled by both the autonomic and somatic nervous systems. The autonomic nervous system acts on an unconscious level and regulates essential bodily functions such as digestion, blood circulation, and breathing. The somatic nervous system is associated with the voluntary control of body movements through skeletal muscles. For example, our breathing continues when we are asleep, and we can also consciously inhale and exhale a deep breath. We cannot, however, actively control the progression of the digestive system or the strength of heart contractions. These continue without any thought process. Prana is the air that we breathe, both unconsciously and consciously. Prana exists everywhere, it is necessary for life, and can be altered from its pervasive, omnipresent state of unconscious, continuous breathing to a consciously controlled state of influence when purposefully drawing in a breath. Just as breath is the crossover between the autonomic and somatic nervous systems, prana can be seen as the link between consciousness and the unconscious.

## AGNI – GOD OF FIRE

*Agni* is the Hindu god of fire. He is thought of as the friend and protector of humanity. The concept of Agni is considered as the source of life, and Ayurvedic practitioners refer to Agni as Gastric Fire. On a physical level, Agni is responsible the transformation of ingested food into substances that the body can absorb and use. Digestive abilities are directly related to the strength of Agni, as are all other chemical reactions and their resulting changes within the body. Agni leads to internal balance and gives the body the strength and power to digest food. Healthy digestion of nutrients leads to correctly absorbed substances and proper assimilation to create strong, healthy tissues. It ensures efficient elimination of waste, helps to fortify healthy gut bacteria, which, in turn helps to prevent disease, and even maintain mental clarity. Agni could be seen as the sum total of the stomach acids and digestive enzymes that activate and maintain a healthy digestive process from ingestion to excretion.

## *AMA – DESTRUCTIVE TOXINS*

On the opposite end of the spectrum from Agni lies *Ama.* In Ayurveda, Ama refers to the accumulation and spread of toxins, which are, ultimately, the major causes of disease. Ama can lead to an impaired metabolism, from which digestive absorption is diminished, resulting in low physical vitality and fatigue. These are primary symptoms of a compromised immune system, which opens the door to an increased risk of infection and disease. In short, Ama is the first domino in a long line of potential ailments, illnesses, and diseases. Whereas Agni reinforces mental clarity, Ama decreases this lucidity. Some of the tangible symptoms of Ama could include bad breath, coated tongue, dull appetite, delicate digestion, fatigue, depression, and difficulty in manifesting intentions. Ama is a foul-smelling, sticky, harmful substance that needs to be completely evacuated from the body.

### SAMPRAPTI – THE SIX STAGES OF DISEASE

According to Ayurveda, the formation of disease follows a relatively straightforward and preventable course of progression, which originates from imbalances in the symbiotic relationship between the mind and the gut, or digestion. The mind is considered to be at the origin of physical imbalances, and the digestive process is manifestation of these physical imbalances. The connection between the gut and the mind is inherent to these principles. The digestive tract is often referred to as "the second brain" of the body. While the brain oversees the functioning of the digestive process via the autonomic nervous system, the enteric nervous system in the digestive tract is responsible for managing not only the digestive process, but also the nearly 100 trillion microbial cells that reside in the gut. These cells are thought to outnumber the body's cells at a ratio of nearly ten to one. The microbial cells found in the gut, called the *microbiota*, are the main influencers for the upkeep and proper functioning of the immune system. The gut is thought to influence the mind's functioning, possibly more so than the brain influences the operation of the digestive tract. There is an intricate, two-way communication system between the brain and the gut. A "gut reaction" refers to an intuitive response to a given situation. When faced with a conundrum, we will often suggest, "Go with your gut," but we rarely hear, "Go with your brain."

The doshas have their physical "seats" in different areas of the digestive tract. Vata is in the colon, Pitta is primarily in the small intestine, and Kapha is primarily in the stomach. A healthy individual is thought to have balance across the three doshas. Imbalance in one of the doshas will manifest itself at the "seat" of that dosha, thus creating digestive symptoms in that area. For example, a Kapha imbalance might be associated with pain soon after eating (stomach), while a Pitta imbalance could manifest through discomfort two to four hours after eating (small intestine), and flatulence or discomfort a long time after eating (colon) might suggest an imbalance in the Vata dosha. Consistent health is inherently linked to the food that we put in to our bodies, which directly influences the digestive process. Thoughts, stress factors, and actions that affect our minds also influence our internal balance and, consequently, digestion.

The six stages of disease progression in Ayurveda are:

*Accumulation* – As one dosha becomes overactive, Ama, the source of disease from the accumulation of toxins, collects in the seat of this overactive dosha.

*Aggravation* – As Ama (toxins) continues to accumulate, symptoms will begin to manifest through the digestive process. These symptoms can range from gas and bloating to sluggish digestion and constipation to acid reflux and burning sensations depending upon the "seat" of the overactive dosha.

*Spread* – When the accumulation of Ama has reached a saturation point at this specific site, it will begin to spread throughout the body. This spread can influence the balance and wellbeing of healthy gut bacteria, through leaky gut syndrome or increased intestinal permeability, and can affect immune function and metabolism.

*Localisation* – Eventually, this spread of Ama will head toward the weaker body tissues. Previously compromised organs, joints, and tissues will be more vulnerable, and the toxins will assimilate into these tissues. The body will attempt to rid itself of the Ama, or toxins. The immune system inevitably attacks the tissues in which these toxins reside. This is the beginning of inflammation.

*Manifestation* – As this process continues over time, the structure and function of the affected tissues or organs will progressively weaken. Signs and symptoms will begin to appear, leading to the eventual diagnosis of a specific disease or illness.

*Complication* – If the condition is not treated as its signs and symptoms are manifested, the condition becomes more complex and begins to create secondary issues. The body's natural repair mechanisms are not able to reverse the dysfunction, which can lead to chronic or permanent conditions. This stage may require surgical interventions or pharmaceutical drug treatment, as the condition has become more widespread and increasingly difficult to manage.

The toxins that begin this process ultimately originate in the mind. They can be in the form of environmental or emotional stress triggers that affect our chemical composition, and they can be in the form of the food that we ingest, which also alters our chemical composition. Perhaps our food intake is in reaction to emotional or environmental factors, or simply due to taste gratification. It all begins with a mental process and decision as to the food that we put into our bodies. The gut-mind connection and the balance of our dosha elements are thus essential to understanding the development of disease as seen through Ayurveda, wherein prevention is the primary source of health care.

### GUNAS – MODES OF EXISTENCE

The impact of elements in life can either be positive, negative, or neutral, and the qualification of these elements can vary over time. Frequently, these qualities exist simultaneously. This is true of people, places, relationships, emotions, objects, and food. In Hindu philosophy, these qualities are called *Gunas*, which can be understood as modes of existence, tendencies, or attributes. The three Gunas are as follows: *Sattva* - goodness, truth, positivity, serenity, and balance. *Rajas* – passion and activity. *Tamas* – destruction, dullness, chaos, and delusion.

In Ayurveda, these concepts help to categorise types of foods and the effects that they have on the body. Sattvic foods might include fruits, ripe vegetables, nuts, seeds, whole grains, seasonal foods, legumes, and non-meat based proteins. A sattvic diet promotes vitality, cleanliness, conscious lifestyle, truth, wisdom, and health. Rajastic foods can provoke mental restlessness. They are neither completely beneficial nor entirely harmful to the body or the mind. These stimulant-related foods include coffee, tea, chocolate, and salt. Tamastic foods can also be thought of as sedative or static foods, which cause or are the result of bodily harm and provoke detrimental stress to physical organs or even entire body systems. Such foods are animal protein, eggs, milk, cheese, processed foods, wheat, sugar and sugar substitutes, as well as chemical preservatives, flavourings, and colourings. The gunas can exist concurrently in the same food. For example, coffee is considered a rajastic or neutral food. It does not possess strict nutritional benefits, nor does it cause inherent harm to the body. It can have sattvic effects, however, if taken in the correct quantity by an athlete prior to a competition or training, as it may help to stimulate the nervous system, delay the physical recognition of fatigue, and increase focus. These are potential positive benefits of coffee. Yet, if one drinks an excessive amount of coffee late at night or on an empty stomach, that coffee can cause insomnia and stomach upset, thus acting as a tamasic food. The same evolution across the gunas can also be seen in fruits, as they go through the ripening process from young and inedible to ripe to eventually overripe and decaying.

These ancient elemental principles can act as modern guidelines in food preparation and consumption, and are living examples of the influence that can be affected over health through nothing more than individual choice. Ayurveda is a complex composite of thoughts and actions. Whether one adheres to Ayurveda as a philosophy or uses it as a health care system is irrelevant. The applied principles of nutrition and the consideration for food that lie within simply offer a bit of insight. Life Knowledge.

### *AYURVEDA – BASIC NUTRITIONAL PRICIPLES*

A few basic principles of Ayurvedic meals are:

*Sattvic* food - primarily whole food plant based, lightly spiced, using no added salt or oil so that you feel refreshed and charged.

Six tastes of Ayurveda – Sweet, sour, salty, pungent, astringent and bitter. Ideally, each meal should contain some representation of each taste.

Food combining – A common cause for indigestion and lack of energy after a meal is more often an imbalance in the combinations and proportions of proteins, carbs and fat. A meal that is balanced in these gives you a boost of energy and vitality.

Right portion – The quantity of food we need varies a little every day based on our daily activity. Eat only as much as you are hungry, and only when you are hungry. For optimum digestion, eat a little less than you desire. Also, try eating in smaller servings rather than one big serving, use smaller plates.

Healthy variety – Meals prepared using a variety of vegetables, roots, greens, fresh herbs, whole grains, lentils, beans, nuts, seeds, dried fruits and spices all provide the complete range of nutrients.

Fresh, local and organic – Eating freshly picked organic seasonal produce from the local farmer's market helps your local economy, helps create a community, and ensures that you get the best, freshest food that is full of all the nutrients.

Cooking tools – It's important to take into consideration the utensils and equipment you cook with. They have to be as natural as possible. Plastic, aluminum, non-stick, anodized cooking utensils may leech toxins into the food so using stainless steel, wood, cast iron, ceramic or glass is the safest.

Seasonal – Eating seasonal fruits and vegetables helps you keep in sync with the cycles of nature. Your body's need for certain food changes according to the seasons of the year. For example, your desire to eat more fresh green, hydrating vegetables in the summer complements the optimum season for these vegetables, just as your desire for dense warming vegetables coincides with their availability and abundance in colder climates. You get the most nutritive value out of a fruit or vegetable when it is eaten in its season.

Do not ingest tamasic foods and ingredients – Avoid food prepared using plastic, aluminum, non-stick and anodized steel utensils; food that is microwaved, canned, or pre-made; food containing processed and refined ingredients like oils, white flour, white sugar, salt and sugar substitutes, corn syrup, preservatives, artificial flavoring, artificial coloring, and is packaged or stored in plastic containers or aluminum.

Cooking method – Cook food only to the extent to make it digestible, while retaining most of its nutritive value. It's important to follow certain processes to retain the nutrients, such as steaming vegetables, soaking and sprouting beans and lentils, and rinsing grains well before cooking.

A special ingredient – Prepare meals for yourself and for others with a positive intention and in a calm environment.

## CHAPTER THREE

*A Brief History, Part II*

When my father found himself on the road of physical decline, he unwittingly charted a straight, downhill route with the wind at his back. The warning lights were ignored with increasing frequency, and he began picking up speed along the way. He refused to acknowledge the inevitability of the other half of the adage about taxes, death. No one gets to choose whether or not he dies. It happens to everyone. Death is the great equalizer. Barring suicide, few people are able to predict or determine the time or place of their passing. Toward the end of his life, my father was seized with a pervasive sense of panic that only released its grip when his body could finally take no more. Death belongs to us all. Each of us is headed there from the day we are born. My father never came to grips with this reality.

My father died at the age of 83. He experienced a relatively long, full existence. He surpassed his own father's life by a whopping 34 years. He enjoyed his grandchildren, and had a loving, committed relationship with my mother for over 60 years. It was never his intention to live forever. He just did not know how to let go, and never truly understood that his life could have ended much differently. Multiple surgical interventions, a desperate and damaging attempt at chemotherapy, and a variety of preventable diseases made the last turns of my father's driving route extremely difficult to negotiate. The road surface was treacherous. He could have chosen an entirely different path to get to where he was going.

My father's approach to life was analytical, yet oddly fatalistic. He relied on science to provide answers, and felt that any specialist in a given field was beyond reproach or question. My father was not a religious man. He did not like systems that relied upon faith. He wanted facts. He reduced life to empirical definitions. Tangible elements were surely easier to understand. He respected his doctors and followed their recommendations as if they were written in stone and delivered from the heavens. My father positioned himself as an authority figure, as a father and a man, and did not like to be questioned. Thus, he did not question other authority figures, especially doctors and surgeons. He received medical opinions as hard fact. There was no room for alternatives. His stubbornness led my father to his death with the same force it had accompanied him with throughout his life.

The final quarter of my father's life was spent dealing with difficult health issues. There were moments of respite, but the root causes of these issues were never addressed, which allowed them to grow. Symptoms were treated, but no real lifestyle changes were ever discussed or made. Life just got slower, more medicated, and more complicated. Sometimes, disease can arrive as a deafening scream, loud and without warning. Usually, however, disease arrives slowly. It is insidious, mostly silent, and virtually invisible. Negative changes occur so slowly that one is almost incapable of even recognising them as changes. Over the course of years or even decades, it continuously tightens the screws until those screws can no longer be removed.

Unchecked disease has a way of presenting the final bill well after the proverbial meal has been eaten. The slow accumulation of poor choices and destructive habits suddenly takes over. For my father, his choices led him into a cul-de-sac of preventable diseases. It took 83 years for these self-inflicted ailments to vanquish him. His final four years were a blinding kaleidoscope of surgical interventions offering no relief, attempted and failed chemical solutions, and intense physical discomfort. My father's zest for life disappeared long before his physical body finally died. He never acknowledged that any of his suffering could have been avoided. Death is one of life's only certainties. The goal is not to avoid death, but rather to prolong a healthy life, free from disease and unnecessary suffering as much as possible. My father's 83 years ended with missing body parts, disease, and emotional and mental confusion. Had my father made a few lifestyle changes when the first warning lights began to flash, his life may have come to an end at the same age even on the same day but perhaps with his body and mind still intact. He could have been spared a tremendous amount of pain and grief.

## CHAPTER FOUR

*The Human Factory*

A s we explore the role of nutrition to prevent disease, it is necessary to understand the basic functioning of the body system that manages the complex process of nutrient absorption. The human digestive system is an intricate network of vital organs that takes the foods we eat and turns them into foods we can use. Everything that we ingest as human beings is utilised, stored, or eliminated by our bodies.

## THE DIGESTIVE PROCESS

The digestive process starts before the food ever hits our mouths. Our brain helps our eyes and nose to get the digestive factory fired up and ready to work by triggering a *salivary response* based on multiple mechanisms of past experience, smell, and anticipated taste. The entire digestive system receives its wake up call. Food then goes into the mouth where it is chewed and broken down into small enough pieces to be swallowed and travel down the *oesophagus* and into the *stomach*.

The stomach has three principal functions, the first of which is to receive the food from the oesophagus. The food is then mixed with digestive acids and enzymes, which further break it down into a mixture that is known as *chyme*. The third function of the stomach is to gradually empty its contents into the small intestine. This emptying process is affected by the nature of the food, primarily its fat and protein content.

The digestive enzymes from the *pancreas* and the *liver* continue the digestive process as the chyme enters the *small intestine*. The autonomic muscular contractions of the digestive system, known as *peristalsis*, push the chyme through the small intestine for further digestion. Absorption of nutrients continues throughout the length of the small intestine (approximately 7 meters, or 22 feet). The waste products of this process include undigested parts of the food, known as fibre, and older cells that have been shed from the walls of the intestine. These materials continue their path into the *colon* (approximately 1.5 meters or 5 feet), where they slowly make their way through to excretion.

The small intestine is the primary site of nutrient absorption. This organ has three distinct segments: the *duodenum*, the *jejunum*, and the *ileum*. Chyme first enters the duodenum from the stomach, where it is exposed to secretions that aid digestion. These secretions include *bile salts* and acids from the liver, which are stored in the *gallbladder* and help to breakdown and digest fats and fat-soluble vitamins (A, D, E, and K). The pancreas also contributes enzymes (*lipase*) that help to digest carbohydrates, fats, and proteins as well as a bicarbonate compound that neutralises the acid from the stomach. The middle part of the small intestine is the jejunum where roughly 90% of nutrient digestion occurs, involving carbohydrates, fats, proteins, vitamins, and minerals. The ileum is the last section of the small intestine. The ileum primarily absorbs water, remaining bile salts, and vitamin B12.

The colon, or large intestine, is the primary site of fluid and *electrolyte* absorption, particularly sodium and potassium. Approximately 1-1.5 litres of fluid are absorbed daily by the colon, which can adapt to 5 litres per day as needed. The colon is the site of stool formation prior to excretion, and also serves to break down and ferment dietary fibre, with the help of healthy gut bacteria, to produce short-chain fatty acids, which can be absorbed and provide added nutrition. Healthy bacteria, which are formed and maintained in the colon, support and ensure proper functioning of the immune system.

The digestive system is highly complex, and performs a multitude of functions. The way in which one of those organs is treated can influence the well-being of all the others. The body is essentially built to survive and will try its best to compensate for shortcomings. This is true throughout the human physical apparatus. It is especially noticeable in the digestive system where the health of the overall system depends upon the health of its individual organs. Their functions are interrelated and interdependent.

## *HORMONAL INFLUENCE – TO EAT OR NOT TO EAT*

The gastrointestinal tract offers a multitude of hormonal influences to the digestive process. These are in addition to and complimentary to the hormones managed by the *endocrine system*, the organs of which have the main responsibilities of regulating and maintaining hormonal balance throughout the body. The various functions of the body's hormones are quite different, yet they all act to keep the body in a functioning equilibrium. Cells responsible for hormonal secretion in the digestive tract are called *enteroendocrine cells*, which do not form glands, but are spread throughout the digestive tract. These cells in the stomach, for example, are responsible for the release of the hormones that control hunger responses. *Ghrelin* stimulates appetite, signals sensations of hunger, promotes fat storage, and increases gastric emptying so as to make room for the next delivery of food into the digestive factory. *Leptin* has an opposite responsibility, which is that of appetite control. Leptin is primarily made and released by adipose cells, which make up the fatty tissue under the skin, known as *adipose tissue*. Leptin helps to regulate energy balance by inhibiting hunger. It lets us know when we feel full during a meal, which should trigger a response to stop eating. These two hormones are simple signals, however, and the human brain can recognise and thus override these signals, allowing us to sometimes push through when we are hungry or to overeat because something simply tastes good. The human body is an amazingly intricate entity, whose functions are extensively and scientifically studied in order to gain an ever-expanding understanding of the chemical responses that interact to make us the species that we are. This basic overview of digestive function will serve as a framework moving forward for understanding how various nutrients are handled by our bodies.

## FUELING THE FACTORY

The foods that our bodies require to maintain proper operation can be placed into two groups, according to how much of that nutrient is needed. These two groups are *macronutrients* and *micronutrients*. Macronutrients are those that we need to consume in large quantities in order to maintain the healthy operation of our bodies. These nutrients include healthy carbs, fats, and proteins. Micronutrients are compounds that are needed in very small quantities, yet play an equally important role in keeping our bodies up and running. Theses compounds are primarily vitamins and minerals. Macronutrients and micronutrients can be derived from a variety of sources, naturally occurring or processed, animal or plant, and the affects they will have on the body can vary dramatically depending upon their origins. When it comes to human nutrition, micronutrient requirements are in amounts generally less than 100 milligrams per day, while macronutrients are required and measured in gram quantities per day. When we refer to a nutrient as "healthy," that precludes the idea that there are some foods that fit the definition for that nutrient, but that are problematic for the human body. As we move forward, let us refer to a healthy nutrient as one that has high nutrient density, and does not cause preventable, foreseeable damage to the human organism. Nutrient density refers to the ratio of nutrients to calories. One should always give preference to foods that contain a high concentration of nutrients, such as macros, vitamins and minerals, fibre, and antioxidants, and avoid foods that are high in calories while providing few inherent benefits to the body, such as processed foods, refined sugars, saturated fats, or any combination of these.

## *MACRONUTRIENTS - HEALTHY CARBOHYDRATES*

*Carbohydrates* are the sugars, starches, and fibres found in fruits, vegetables, grains, and some dairy products. Carbohydrate consumption is essential for optimal health. The *recommended daily amount (RDA)* of carbohydrate consumption for an adult human is

135 grams, although this may vary from person to person depending upon his or her individual object-ives, including weight loss or sports performance. Carb intake for most people should be around sixty-five per cent of total daily calorie intake. One gram of carbohydrates equals roughly four calories.

Carbohydrates are the essential source of fuel for the central nervous system and energy for muscle move-ment. The presence of ingested and subsequently stored carbs in the body prevents protein from being used as a primary source of energy, thus preserving muscle tone and strength. Carbohydrates are also an important factor in proper brain function, as they can influence memory and mood. There are two types of carbs: simple and complex. *Simple carbohy-drates* contain either just one sugar (*monosaccharides*) or two sugars (*disaccharides*). *Fructose* (fruits) and gal-actose (dairy products) are monosaccahrides, while *sucrose* (table sugar), *lactose* (also in dairy products), and *maltose* (beer and some vegetables) are disac-charides. Simple carbs can also present themselves in the forms of candy, soda, and syrups, which are highly processed, contain no vitamins, minerals, or dietary fibre. These are essentially empty calories and can easily lead to weight gain and a host of other ailments. *Complex carbohydrates* have three or more sugars (*polysaccharides*), and include starchy foods, such as beans, peas, lentils, potatoes, parsnips, and whole grain cereals. Simple carbs are digested more quickly than complex carbs, and are thus used for short bursts of energy. Simple carbs can cause spikes in blood sugar levels, with sugar highs and inevitable crashes, while complex carbs provide more sustained energy. Carbohydrates should be taken in from naturally occurring sources like fruits, vegetables, and whole grains, rather then processed and packaged foods.

The body breaks down carbohydrates into smaller units of sugar, such as glucose and fructose. These smaller units are absorbed by the small intestine, where they then enter the bloodstream and travel to the liver. The liver converts all of these sugars into glucose, which is carried through the bloodstream — accompanied by insulin to continuously regulate the level of blood glucose — and converted into energy for basic body functioning and physical activity.

If the glucose is not immediately needed for energy, the body can store up to 2,000 calories of it in the liver and skeletal muscles in the form of *glycogen*. Once these glycogen stores are full, carbohydrates are stored as fat. The body will first seek out the glycogen stored in the muscles. Once these levels are depleted, the glycogen stored in the liver will be solicited and used for energy. When there is no longer any available glycogen to be used as fuel, the body will then turn to fat as its source of energy. The human body can only store carbohydrate energy (glycogen) for a short time, one or two days, while fat is stored on a long-term basis. When carbohydrates are scarce, the body runs mainly on fats. If energy needs exceed those provided by fats in the diet, the body must liquidate some of its fat tissue for energy.

### MACRONUTRIENTS - HEALTHY FATS

As with carbohydrates, there are various types of *fats*. Some are necessary and beneficial while others have a negative, detrimental effect on the body. As carbohydrates should provide approximately sixty-five per cent of daily calorie intake, fats should provide around twenty per cent. The different types of fats are identified by their composition. Fats are essentially composed of *glycerol* and *fatty acids*. It is the chemical configuration of their carbon bonds that determines into which category of fats they fall, and how these fats are dealt with in the body.

The four types of fats found in foods are *saturated, monounsaturated, polyunsaturated,* and *trans fats*. Saturated fats are those found in most animal products, including meat, butter, and cheese, as well as coconut and palm oil. These are high in fat, contain no dietary fibre, and have been shown to increase cholesterol levels. Monounsaturated fats can be found in avocados and olives. These fats help to protect the heart and reduce insulin sensitivity, fat storage, and weight loss. Polyunsaturated fats, found in a variety of nuts and seeds, include Omega 3 and Omega 6 compounds, which both have benefits for the human body.

Omega 3's reduce inflammation, support healthy hormone levels and cell membranes. Omega 6's support healthy brain and muscle function, but promote inflammation in the body. A health-promoting ratio of Omega 6 to Omega 3 would be below 4:1. Most Western diets have a ratio of 15:1 or higher. Corn, soybean, safflower, cottonseed, grapeseed and sunflower oils are all contain high amounts of omega 6's and are not stable. This means any food that is fried, baked, or microwaved using these oils will oxidize and create an inflammatory response in the body.

Trans fats are highly processed vegetable oils and should be avoided entirely. They are present in cookies, cakes, biscuits, doughnuts, crackers, margarine, microwave popcorn, fried fast foods, and frozen pizza. Harvard University's *The Nutrition Source* states the following with regard to trans fats: "*It is a by-product of a process called hydrogenation that is used to turn healthy oils into solids and to prevent them from becoming rancid. When vegetable oil is heated in the presence of hydrogen and a heavy-metal catalyst such as palladium, hydrogen atoms are added to the carbon chain. This turns oils into solids. It also makes healthy vegetable oils more like not-so-healthy saturated fats. On food label ingredient lists, this manufactured substance is typically listed as 'partially hydrogenated oil.'*"

As a general rule, saturated and trans fats should be avoided, as they are associated with cardiovascular disease, increased risk of stroke, high cholesterol levels, and various forms of cancer, including breast, colorectal, ovarian, and prostate cancer. While some nut and seed oils may hold potential health benefits, it is necessary to remember that all oils are processed. Chemically extracted oil from a whole food no longer contains the vast quantity of micronutrients, fibers, and flavanoids that give that food its power. Fragmented foods contain little more than empty calories.

Health promoting fats are naturally occurring in plant foods. Nuts, seeds, olives, and avocados are good sources of healthy fats, Omega 3's, and Omega 6's. Fats that exist in these foods are not processed, and also come with other beneficial compounds, such as fibre, which helps with the proper absorption of these fats, and antioxidants, which fight inflammation and the premature aging of tissues. Consumption of whole foods will provide greater benefits than the extracted or processed elements of these whole foods. A holistic, inclusive outlook toward what we eat should be similar to the way a holistic practitioner might regard his or her patient: the sum of the individual parts is less than the whole.

### *MACRONUTRIENTS - PROTEINS*

*Proteins* consist of a variety of amino acids. Some of these amino acids are made in the body, while others, known as *essential amino acids*, must be obtained through the food we eat. There are twenty different types of amino acids that can be combined to form a protein. The sequence of amino acids determines the shape and function of the protein that they bind together to create. Protein functions include antibody support, enzyme creation for chemical reactions within cells, messenger cells that acts as communicators between different cells, tissues, and organs, a structural component which allows the body to move, and transport/storage that bind and carry atoms and small molecules throughout the body. Protein is considered a foundational element to life and is found in every cell of the body.

The recommended daily amount of protein intake is 0.8 grams per kilogram of body weight, and should constitute approximately fifteen per cent of total daily calorie intake. Individual daily intake targets of protein may vary for professional athletes who could increase the "per kilogram of body weight" amount from 0.8 to somewhere between 1.1 to 1.7 grams per kilo of body weight. Anything over 2.0 is considered excessive and may present a negative impact on overall health. Proteins, and the amino acids that compose them, are the building blocks of skeletal muscle, and can also be used as an energy source by the body when carbohydrates and fats are not available. If carbohydrate intake or stores are insufficient, and fats are unavailable, the body will consume protein for fuel. This is problematic, however, because the body needs protein to build and maintain muscle tone and strength. Using protein instead of carbohydrates or fats for fuel also puts increased stress on the *kidneys*, leading to possible inflammation and the eventual passage of painful by-products, such as *kidney stones*, in the urine.

All proteins are not created equal. Again, it is important to select foods that have a high nutrient density and that are not known to be detrimental or restrictive to optimal health. A protein is considered "complete" when it contains all nine of the essential amino acids that we need to get from our diet, and which are necessary for proper functioning of the body. Animal proteins from meat and eggs are complete. Due to their high levels of saturated fats and complete absence of dietary fibre, however, animal proteins are also known to largely contribute to myriad diseases, such as cardiovascular disease, blood vessel dysfunction, coronary heart disease, stroke, Type-2 diabetes, high cholesterol, and obesity. Animal proteins also have an acidifying effect on the body, which promotes inflammation. In order to neutralise the acidic pH levels, the parathyroid gland signals the bones to release calcium to re-establish a more alkaline state in the body, thus potentially weakening the bones and creating favourable conditions for the onset of osteoporosis. Plant proteins include beans, nuts, whole grains, and vegetables. Some plant proteins are complete (quinoa, hemp, soy, brown rice, and pumpkin), yet if some sources are not complete, they simply need to be combined with other complimentary plant protein sources so as to offer the body the complete panel of the nine essential amino acids. Plant proteins are free from saturated fats and contain dietary fibre, as well as a multitude of antioxidant compounds, which are preventative and curative for the body. It is important to choose your protein sources, and to remember that excessive protein intake can be detrimental to optimal health.

Macronutrients are the primary sources of energy and are thus required in large amounts. They constitute the totality of the food we eat. Just as we saw the importance of taking the whole person into account for a holistic approach to the health, it is equally important to see the foods we eat as whole units. Most of the food items we eat will contain some combination of all macronutrients. They do not generally exist as isolated elements. The balance of these elements within each food item is important to recognise, and it is equally essential to target for the optimal ratios of macronutrients throughout the day. An avocado, for example, might contain around 75% healthy fat, 20% carbohydrates, and 5% protein. Avocado is clearly a "fat dominant" food, yet still contains carbs and protein. Eating a varied selection of whole plant foods can ensure a correct balance of nutritional intake. The suggested percentage of each macronutrient is flexible. Balance is, again, the most important factor when choosing what you eat. This allows for a variety of taste and flavours, and ensures that you are offering a wide selection of nutrients to your body.

## *INTERACTION OF THE ELEMENTS*

Micronutrients are those nutrients that the human body requires in small amounts, yet are essential for its proper functioning. These are *vitamins* and *minerals*, and are considered essential nutrients due to the fact that the human body cannot manufacture enough of them on its own. These compounds must therefore be ingested via the food that we choose to eat. Micronutrients are necessary compounds in and of themselves; they can also interact in various ways so as to enhance, encourage, and enrich other micronutrients that they encounter. The reverse is also true, however, as some of these compounds can actually inhibit and nullify the absorption and benefits of other micronutrients. For example, vitamin D allows your body to extract and use calcium from food sources travelling through your intestine, rather than requiring the body to leach the necessary calcium for the bones. Inversely, vitamin C can inhibit assimilation of the essential mineral copper. One must be conscious of maintaining a healthy balance of these naturally occurring compounds, as deficiency or excessive supplementation can create dangerous chemical imbalances for which the body's systems will have to compensate.

## *MICRONUTRIENTS – VITAMINS*

Vitamins can be separated into water-soluble and fat-soluble, while minerals can be identified as either *major minerals* or *trace minerals*. Water-soluble vitamins are found in the watery portions of fruits and vegetables, and are readily absorbed into the bloodstream during digestion of these foods. The kidneys act as filters, eliminating excess amounts of these vitamins through the urine. *Water-soluble vitamins* include the B-complex vitamins. These include biotin (vitamin B7), folic acid (folate, vitamin B9), Niacin (vitamin B3), pantothenic acid (vitamin B5), riboflavin (vitamin B2), and vitamins B6 and B12. Vitamin C is also a water-soluble compound. Basically, these vitamins are responsible for the production and release of energy from foods, building protein and cells, and the formation of collagen. Whereas water-soluble vitamins are directly absorbed into the bloodstream to perform their roles, fat-soluble vitamins enter the body through lymph channels in the intestine. Many of these vitamins travel through the body only under escort by proteins that act as carriers. Fat-soluble compounds are stored by the body in its fatty tissues and in the liver, and are held there until needed, thus working as a sort of time-release micronutrient. *Fat-soluble vitamins* include vitamins A, D, E, and K, and their main functions are to build bones, protect vision, interact favourably, and protect the body.

## MICRONUTRIENTS – MAJOR MINERALS

Major minerals are as crucial to the body as are trace minerals. The body simply stores and requires them in a greater amount.

The major minerals are:

*Calcium (C)*

*Chloride (Cl)*

*Magnesium (Mg)*

*Phosphorus (P)*

*Potassium (K)*

*Sodium (Na)*

*Sulfur (S)*

Major minerals travel through the body and are absorbed in various ways. Potassium is rapidly absorbed into the bloodstream, much like a water-soluble vitamin, whereas calcium requires a carrier for transport and absorption, much like a fat-soluble vitamin. Their key tasks include water, or *electrolyte*, balance (sodium, chloride, and potassium), maintenance of healthy bones (calcium, phosphorus, and magnesium), and stabilisation of protein structure, including hair, skin, and nails (sulphur). Electrolytes, as their name implies, are responsible for the electrical impulses that flow through our cells and ensure proper body functioning. Their imbalance can have far-reaching negative consequences for health. Imbalances in these compounds are usually due to over-loads from unbalanced supplementation or, in certain cases, depletion, rather than directly from food sources.

### MICRONUTRIENTS – TRACE MINERALS

Trace minerals include:

*Chromium (Cr)*

*Copper (Cu)*

*Fluorine (F)*

*Iodine (I)*

*Iron (Fe)*

*Manganese (Mn)*

*Molybdenum (Mo)*

*Selenium (Se)*

*Zinc* (Zn)

These compounds carry out a wide variety of tasks directly related to optimal body function. They help to prevent damage to body cells, are foundational elements in the formation of key enzymes, and can enhance the activity of these enzymes. Whereas some major minerals, like calcium and phosphorus, may account for up to a half a kilo each of overall body weight, all trace minerals combined may only amount to the equivalent of a couple of eye droppers.

Macronutrients are the compounds that help to regulate balance in our bodies and to ensure the proper functioning of cells, organs, and systems. They can be found easily by eating quality fruits and vegetables on a regular basis. The nutrition that we get from whole, naturally occurring foods is highest when those foods are organic, local, fresh, and seasonal. Pesticides and long transport time from farm to market can diminish, damage, and destroy certain nutrients in food. Clearly, it is better to eat a fruit that has ripened with minimal chemical interference on the tree in relatively local surroundings rather one that has been picked prematurely and ripens over days or weeks of transport time from a distant land. A well-rounded diet of whole, naturally occurring foods helps to ensure adequate consumption and balance of macronutrients as well as micronutrients.

## CHAPTER FIVE

*The Endocrine System*

L ife Knowledge. There is more to each of us than biological explanations, physiological func- tions, anatomical descriptions, and environ- mental conditions. We are complex, emotional beings. We cannot be studied or understood in an empirical manner. No two people will interpret or react to the same event - physically, emotionally, or mentally - in exactly the same way. All factors must be considered, and even those factors are on a mov- ing timeline. Reductive analysis will not help. We are like a delicious bowl of homemade soup. All of the ingredients have a unique and discernible flavour, yet, when cooked together, these flavours change, influence one another, and come together to cre- ate a new flavour. The soup is always different, and every spoonful of the same soup is different because the temperature has changed, our perceptions have adjusted, and our recognition of the taste of the first spoonful alters our notion of the next spoonful. Human beings are in constant flux. We are living, breathing examples of the concept of perpetual change.

## HORMONES AND BALANCE

There is one complex, physical system of human organs that embodies this concept through its functions: the endocrine system. This collection of separate yet interconnected organs and functions has the continuously evolving task of maintaining physical, emotional, and psychological balance within each person. The endocrine organs, or glands, receive information from various sources, ranging from nutritional input to environmental stresses and pleasures to internally perceived emotions to physical threats coming from within the body itself. Each organ interprets the information it has received, and reacts by excreting specific hormones into the bloodstream in an attempt to restore balance.

An *endocrine gland* is a ductless gland that releases a substance directly into the bloodstream, whereas an exocrine gland must secrete via a duct, or passageway. The pancreas is an example of a gland with both exocrine and endocrine functions. As we saw earlier, the pancreas releases digestive enzymes into the gastrointestinal tract via a duct, while it is also responsible for insulin and glucagon, the hormones that regulate blood glucose levels, which are excreted directly into the bloodstream. The glands of the endocrine system produce hormones that help to regulate metabolism, growth and development, tissue function, sexual function, reproduction, sleep, and mood, amongst other functions. The major endocrine glands, from lowest physical location to highest, and their corresponding hormones include:

**Gonads** – This term refers to the *ovaries*, the female reproductive organ, and *testes*, the male counterpart. The ovaries produce *progesterone* and *oestrogen*. The testes are responsible for the production of *testosterone*.

**Adrenal Glands** – These glands are small structures attached to the top of each kidney. The adrenal cortex produce *glucocorticoids*, primarily *cortisol*, which acts to reduce inflammation and stimulate immune response, *mineralocorticoids*, including *aldosterone,* which helps to regulate and maintain salt and water levels in the body, which, in turn, regulates blood pressure. The adrenal medulla produces *adrenalin*, *noradrenelin*, and small amounts of *dopamine.* These hormones are responsible for the *fight or flight response*, and are the stress regulators in the body.

**Pancreas** – The pancreas is located behind the stomach. It is an exocrine gland as well as an endocrine gland, meaning that it is both ducted and ductless. In its endocrine function, the pancreas produces and regulates the hormones *glucagon*, which raises blood glucose levels when they are low, and *insulin*, which lowers blood glucose levels. Insulin triggers the absorption of glucose from the blood into cells, where it is added to glycogen molecules for storage. The pancreas is a crucial organ for the mediation of blood glucose levels.

**Thymus** – The thymus is the primary specialised lymphoid organ of the immune system, and is part of the *lymphatic system*, as well as the endocrine system. It is located behind the sternum and between the lungs. It produces *T-lymphocytes* and *thymosin* that help to protect the body from *pathogens*. The thymus is large during infancy, when the human organism is in its most fragile state, and subsequently and continuously diminishes in size after puberty. Its function, however, remains as the primary reactor to the immune system throughout the duration of a person's life.

**Thyroid Gland** – This gland is located in the neck, toward the front of the *larynx*. It produces *thyroxin*, which regulates metabolic rate, and *calcitonin*, which regulates the uptake of calcium to the bones.

**Parathyroid Glands** – The parathyroid glands are tiny glands located directly behind the thyroid gland. The task of these glands is to regulate calcium *homeostasis* in the blood. They produce *parathyroid hormone (PTH)*, which raises blood calcium levels by breaking down bone and causing calcium release by stimulating the body's ability to absorb calcium from food, and by increasing the kidney's ability to hold on to calcium that would otherwise be excreted in the urine. They ensure proper and constant calcium levels, which are crucial for vital body functions.

**Pituitary Gland** – This gland is part of the brain, and is known as the Master Gland. The pituitary gland, which is approximately the size of a pea, regulates *growth hormones* and *oxytocin,* amongst many others, which travel throughout the body, directing certain processes or stimulating other glands to produce other hormones. *(Anne Klibanski, MD and Nicholas Tritos, MD).*

**Pineal Gland** – The pineal gland is located in the back of the brain of all animals with backbones. It produces *melatonin*, which regulates sleep patterns in both *circadian* and seasonal cycles. The shape of this gland resembles a pinecone, hence its name, and also influences the pituitary gland. French philosopher, Réné Descartes, referred to the pineal gland as "the seat of the soul."

**Hypothalamus** – The hypothalamus is a part of the brain and is located near the pituitary gland. It has many functions, such as regulating body temperature, maintaining daily physiological cycles, controlling appetite, managing sexual behaviour, and recognising emotional responses, amongst others. It releases numerous hormones, including *oxytocin*, which influences many behaviours and emotions, such as sexual arousal, trust, recognition, and maternal behaviour, as well as childbirth and lactation. *(Jill Seladi-Schulman PhD, Seunggu Han, MD)*

The endocrine system is constantly evaluating and adjusting hormonal levels to maintain balance. It is constantly in a state of movement to make the necessary shifts and changes to keep a person in an optimal state of equilibrium. The interaction of these glands and the hormones that they produce is intricate and fragile. The capacity for adjustment to compensate for imbalance is robust; repeated or continued abuse of the system, however, will eventually result in a system breakdown.

### STRESS – TRIGGERS AND RESPONSES

Since the endocrine system is constantly responding, even to subtle input like the sound of someone shouting in the street outside, the organs of this system are often hardest hit by threats or discomforts in our environment. It is also the first system to respond to any negative thoughts or actions. The endocrine system is a sort of internal bodyguard, physically, mentally, and emotionally. Endocrine imbalances can arise from within the thoughts of the individual as well as from his or her outside environment. Questioning and criticizing the self, making natural responses "wrong," or living in an environment where one feels under threat, at any level, are all factors that can affect the endocrine system. Physical threat can come from outside sources, just as it can come from body's reactions to poor nutritional habits and choices, which the body's systems will inevitably receive as a threat.

Stress triggers are rampant throughout the course of daily life, though very few of these are truly or immediately life-threatening. The physical and chemical reactions to environmental stress factors, however, do not differentiate levels of danger. If left unchecked, this input can create a continual hormonal stress reaction. These physical stress factors can arise from environment, nutrition, and lifestyle. Just as poor food choices can have a detrimental impact on the endocrine system, healthy food choices can prevent and even reverse damage to these sensitive organs. Certain foods are known to have a negative effect on the human body; they have been identified as promoters of disease, creators of negative imbalance, and triggers of chronic inflammation. Each person is solely responsible for that which he or she chooses to eat. Nutritional choices are amongst the few potential and known stress factors for the human body that can be almost completely controlled by the individual. It is rare to see someone being force fed a hamburger, fries, and a milkshake against his will. The choice to promote and ensure health through food is within reach of each individual.

The complexity of the endocrine system and the health of its organs can be influenced by personal choices. A well-rounded, whole food plant based lifestyle can help to ensure the wellbeing of this system, thus facilitating your body's task of maintaining balance and optimal health. By offering your body a diet rich in nutrient dense food, antioxidants, and naturally occurring dietary fiber, you can support the functions that keep it in balance. Foods to seek include fresh, organic fruits and vegetables, whole grains, healthy fats, and quality plant proteins. Inversely, food choices that provide the body with chemicals, pesticides, preservatives, and high amounts of fats and sugars will have a markedly detrimental impact on overall health. Foods to avoid include all processed foods, refined sugar, trans fats, all GMO foods, wheat, and animal products. Toxins are stored in fat cells, so eating animal fat, meat and dairy, releases any ingested toxins, ranging from growth hormones to antibiotics to steroids, into the human body.

Lifestyle choices can also favor or endanger the endocrine system. Many environmental factors are beyond our realm of direct control, and, while we may not be able to alter these factors, we can certainly influence the way in which they are received by our minds and bodies. Lifestyle choices that ensure endocrine health can include regular exercise, yoga and meditation, efforts toward mental clarity with oneself and others, and reframing situations to strive for a more positive outlook. Risk factors for the endocrine organs can include mental and emotional confusion, detrimental physical choices, such as the consumption of alcohol, cigarettes, and drugs, stress and stressful situations, and eating and drinking from plastic containers, as toxins from plastic can leach into the food that we consume. BPA and other plastic by-products are known to be endocrine disruptors as they mimic hormonal activity and can provoke unwanted and dangerous reactions. All of these factors can have profound effects on the body's ability to rectify the imbalances that they create.

The fragility of the endocrine system is matched only by its robust and comprehensive nature of functioning. Imbalances are inherent to the human organism; however, we can directly influence and affect the gravity, frequency, and longevity of these imbalances through personal nutritional and lifestyle choices. Buddha has been credited with stating, "To keep the body in good health is a duty... Otherwise we shall not be able to keep our mind strong and clear." The connection between body and mind is intricate and undeniable. If the body is in difficulty, the mind will struggle as a result. Inversely, if we do everything in our control to nurture and maintain our physical beings, we shall help all aspects of the mental, intellectual, and emotional self to thrive. We can directly influence the health of our bodies through exercise and nutrition, thus cutting down the workload of the balancing organs of the endocrine system.

## CHAPTER SIX

*A Brief History, Part III*

During the final years of my father's life, when his physical health was hurtling into the irreversible vortex of progressive disease and invasive medical interventions, my mother made the choice to become his primary caretaker. At that time, they had been inseparable partners for sixty years. My mother's choice was logical and committed. My father needed care and she was going to be the one to provide it. As much as my father trusted and admired the medical profession, my mother was reticent and unimpressed by medical doctors. She respected my father's wishes, however, and followed their medical directives as best she could.

My mother had been astounded at the doctor's suggestion to proceed with an intrusive and compromising ileostomy, which would remove the lower portion of my father's entire digestive tract. Given the advanced nature of my father's multiple diseases, his then current weakened state, and, above all, his advanced age, my mother had not expected major surgery as a worthy option. He was not a young man with many years of life before him. He was 82 years old at the time, and had been accumulating major illnesses for the past few years. The doctor presented my father with the option of this medical intervention, which he said might prolong my father's life for as long as a few months to a year. The doctor was simply doing his due diligence by presenting medical solutions. He was there to present options, not to give advice about which option to select, nor did he address the potential decrease in quality of life that might ensue. He was a surgeon who explained the surgery, and how it might offer a solution to an existing problem. As shocked as my mother had been at the doctor's recommendation for surgery, she was equally as saddened by my father's decision to move forward with it. She had expected my father to come to grips with his own mortality, and to spare himself and his family some excruciatingly difficult final months. My mother knew my father better than anyone however, and this decision did not come as much of a surprise to her.

The daily stress of dealing with seemingly endless amounts of paperwork from Medicare, Medicaid, the hospital, and private health insurance, was overwhelming to my mother not to mention the bank and credit card statements. She had never paid a bill or handled even the smallest amount of administrative paperwork. My father had always dealt with these things and now he was too sick to handle them. My mother stepped up as best she could with the help of her family, which, for the most part, was scattered in different states and distant countries. Between the quagmire of confusing administrative obligations and the complicated caretaking of my father, my mother was well beyond her comfort level. Amongst all of this, she was also grieving for a soon-to-be lost partner of sixty years. My father was still physically alive, but the flame, which had defined him as a man, had long been extinguished.

When my father exhaled his final breath, my mother was naturally distraught, yet saw this as some sort of deliverance from the intense difficulties that had come to define his life. His inability to acknowledge his own mortality made the end of his life sad, complicated, and filled with dread. My father died peacefully, surrounded by his family, in a hospital bed. He wanted to have nurses and doctors around him. My mother had put her own emotions aside during her time as caretaker. She had managed my father to the best of her ability. There had been no room to anticipate grief or loss. When my father died, however, grief came rushing over her like a great tidal wave capable of submerging villages. She was never truly able to get her head above water again.

My mother was a relatively healthy woman, whose only medical obligation was to monitor her blood pressure every two days and remember to take her medicine, which she did with great diligence. During my father's illness, she had slightly neglected her own nutrition. My mother struggled with the intimate details of my father's ileostomy, and lost most of her appetite and overall desire for food. She tried to push through the grief and stress of my father's final few years, but she was deeply saddened. She had always been a joyous, communicative woman who found wonderment in every detail of life, but after my father's death, everything changed. My mother died suddenly, of natural causes, nine months after my father passed. She showed no signs of physical illness. There were no hospitals, no doctors, no interventions, and no medication.

The stress that had become an integral part of my mother's life was an undeniable culprit for her death. She had been pushed well past her comfort levels, and the toll was a heavy one to pay. The grief of a profound loss only added to her downward spiral. It became clear that stress had essentially eaten away the few resources that my mother still had left within her. Her physical body was no longer able to do its job. It could ne longer compensate for the damage that had been inflicted from difficult life conditions. She was finally overcome.

## CHAPTER SEVEN

## Lifestyle: Causes and Effects

The trickle down effects of stress on the body can be far reaching. The human organism strives for balance at all times. Emotional, mental, and physical equilibrium is what allows us to move forward from day to day. This balance can be adversely affected by choices, positive and negative, on a vast scale.

### TELOMERES – DNA PROTECTION

Prolonged stress of any kind can eventually even damage our DNA, which holds the genetic information of the cells of our body. Protective sheaths, called *telomeres*, cover the DNA potion of the stem cells that are responsible for cell division and renewal. Healthy telomeres are long, and keep the DNA intact so that cell division can proceed smoothly, without anomalies. If a cell's telomeres become too short, they send signals out that put a stop to the division of that cell. This means that the cell cannot renew itself, and, as with anything that cannot renew itself, it becomes old and stagnant. The DNA of old cells does not communicate its information as readily or accurately, and thus cannot respond normally to stresses. Over time, stress - physical or psychological - wears down the telomeres, and creates very favorable conditions for cell dysfunction and eventual disease. (*The Telomere Effect by Elizabeth Balckburn, PhD and Elissa Epal, PhD*)

## PERSONAL CHOICES - POSITIVE OR NEGATIVE

This is a microscopic look into the holistic person, so let's step back to see what this really means. Essentially, the actions that we fulfill during our lives can either be positive or negative. They can be either enriching or damaging. These actions include the foods we eat, the relationships we maintain, the jobs we do, the hobbies and sports we practice, and virtually every other aspect of our lives. Of course, not every person makes the best decisions all the time. We all have made, make, and will continue to make mistakes throughout our lives. Poor choices are an integral part of the human experience. Trial and error is a viable way of learning from our mistakes, and attempting to avoid repeating them. The way we treat the world directly affects what happens within our holistic, integrative person. Our bodies are resilient and forgiving. By altering detrimental choices, we are able to rectify damaging actions. Our bodies will thank us and forgive us if we are able to heed the warning lights that will inevitably flash for each of us at some point in our lives. Balance will thus be easier to achieve and maintain.

The internal state of the human body can be measured using a *pH* scale, which measures the acidity level of our body on a scale from 1 to 14, with 1 being the most acidic and 14 the most basic, or alkaline. Either of the extremes can be dangerous. It can be useful to measure your pH level so as to understand the internal state of affairs and make any necessary changes to ensure proper balance. Imagine a *pH* test for our life choices. Are we doing everything that is within our realm of control to ensure healthy balance and to promote personal longevity, or are we knowingly or unwittingly making choices that increase the "extreme" parts of our lives, and thus shortening the proverbial and literal telomeres that protect the very essence of who we are?

### *CHOOSING HEALTH*

A whole food plant based lifestyle emphasizes a large variety of nutrition that comes from naturally occurring whole foods. It does not involve animal products, including meat of any kind, fish, dairy, or eggs. Heavily processed foods of any kind are not included in a whole food plant based lifestyle, either. These foods include refined grain products, such as white rice and white flour, refined sugars and artificial sweeteners, such as table sugar or high fructose corn syrup, and processed fats, including oils. This may seem like a draconian set of conditions as to the foods that we should eat and the foods that we should avoid. Certainly, it may require some discipline and strong will to break away from past, socially nurtured habits; however, if these habits are proven pathways to disease and chronic health problems, then perhaps they deserve to be abandoned. The benefits of a whole food plant based lifestyle are far reaching, as they directly affect physical and mental health, undeniably impact the issues of global warming and world hunger, and offer consideration of ethical questions that are increasingly important to the well being of not just the individual, but to the world's population as a whole.

A whole food plant based lifestyle enhances the existence of other sentient beings, and decreases one's risk of life-threatening physical ailments and chronic diseases. The food that one puts in his or her body is one of the fundamental choices that an individual can make with regard to overall health. Selecting foods that either work for you or against you is up to each person. Free will. Free choice. Certain foods do not only prevent disease, they can also help to cure disease. Making informed food choices is a major lifestyle step toward self-determination.

A person's level of health has a direct correlation with what that person puts into his or her body. Foods can be disease preventing or disease promoting. Remember the gunas from Ayurveda: sattvic, rajastic, or tamasic. Positive, neutral, or negative. The knowledge of which is which, and the potential or proven impacts that either can have on your health is essential to taking responsibility for eventual outcomes. Gaining control of your health is an empowering action that is well within reach. It starts with the foods you choose, as these are the basic elements that keep you going throughout the day, and throughout your life.

## *BODY WEIGHT AND CALORIES*

Weight control is a concern that affects a vast amount of people. The Obesity Medicine Association's definition of obesity is "a chronic, relapsing, multifactorial, neurobehavioral disease, wherein an increase in body fat promotes adipose tissue dysfunction and abnormal fat mass physical forces, resulting in adverse metabolic, biomechanical, and psychosocial health consequences." *Encylopedia Britannica* explains *obesity* as "excessive accumulation of body fat, usually caused by the consumption of more calories than the body can use. The excess calories are then stored as fat, or adipose tissue." Obesity is generally defined as an increase in body weight that is greater than 20% of that individual's ideal body weight according to a calculation known as Body Mass Index (BMI). BMI, used by *Centres for Disease Control and Prevention* and the *World Health Organisation*, is a person's weight in kilograms divided by his height squared in meters. This number takes into account height, weight, age, and gender. It is not a direct measure of actual fat in the body, but rather a parallel measure to help identify individuals as underweight, healthy weight, overweight, or obese. For example, an individual with a BMI of 30 or more is considered to be obese.

## OBESITY – THE INTERNAL TIMEBOMB

A few statistics from the World Health Organization, published in February 2018:

- Worldwide obesity has nearly tripled since 1975.

- In 2016, more than 1.9 billion adults, 18 years and older, were overweight. Of these over 650 million were obese.

- 39% of adults aged 18 years and over were overweight in 2016, and 13% were obese.

- Most of the world's population live in countries where overweight and obesity kills more people than underweight.

- 41 million children under the age of 5 were overweight or obese in 2016.

- Over 340 million children and adolescents aged 5-19 were overweight or obese in 2016.

- Obesity is preventable.

Obesity is directly linked to an increased frequency in non-communicable and preventable diseases, such as heart disease, stroke, osteoarthritis, Type-2 diabetes, and various forms of cancer, including endometrial (uterus), breast, ovarian, prostate, liver, gallbladder, kidney, and colon. Many of these same diseases are also carry a direct link to the consumption of animal products. Whole food plant based nutritional choices do not include animal products and processed foods, which are the highest in saturated fats and other damaging substances that can contribute to the accumulated fat and excess calories that lead to obesity.

### CALORIES – NOT ALL ARE CREATED EQUAL

*Cambridge English Dictionary* defines a *calorie* as "a unit of energy, often used as a unit of measurement of the amount of energy that food provides when eaten and digested." The scientifically precise term and definition is *kilocalorie*, which represents the amount of energy required to raise the temperature of a liter of water by one degree Celsius. When thought of as an empirical unit of food energy, all calories should be equivalent to the body. Each person needs a relatively simple to calculate number of calories in order to properly function through the day. The number of calories may vary depending upon age, gender, and activity level. All calories, however, are not created equal.

It is virtually impossible to overeat plant-based foods, as these are generally high in nutrient density and relatively low in calories. One will get a feeling of *satiety*, or fullness, before excessive calorie intake occurs. For example, 300 grams of broccoli would fill you up, is very high in nutrients, and contains only 100 calories. One will get a feeling of fullness due to volume before excess calorie intake sets in.

Processed foods, however, are quite the opposite. Potato chips, for example, are small and possess virtually zero nutritional attributes. They are extremely high in calories, saturated fat and salt, however, and they do not fill you up. It is easy to overeat this type of food, and to have a huge level of calories ingested without ever feeling fullness, or satiety. Calories do not fill you up; nutrients and food volume give you the feeling of satiety.

It is slightly different, although no less detrimental, for meats and cheeses. 300 grams of animal-based food might contain up to ten times the number of calories as that same 300 grams of broccoli, 1,000 calories compared to 100. Animal foods and their by-products are also very high in fat and cholesterol, thus generally high in calories, and possess no dietary fibre at all, which translates to slower, heavier digestion and excess absorption and storage of unneeded saturated fat. Even small amounts of these foods will dramatically increase calorie intake, in addition to the numerous long-term detrimental effects that they have on the human body, including inflammation, insulin resistance, obesity, and chronic disease.

A whole food plant-based diet will help to regulate body weight without counting calories, as it is difficult to overeat whole grains, nuts, seeds, vegetables, and fruits. The combination of these naturally occurring foods, unprocessed and free from animal products, along with daily exercise are crucial to naturally allowing the body to find and maintain its proper weight.

## CHAPTER EIGHT

*You Are What You Eat*

*D*ietary fiber is a key component to disease prevention. By including foods that are high in
fiber, you can reduce the risk of hemorrhoids,
diverticulitis, colorectal cancer, high blood pressure,
high cholesterol, chronic inflammation, Type-2 diabetes, and irregular bowel movements. Also, high
fiber foods can help to stabilize and maintain optimal weight. Unlike macro and micronutrients, which
are broken down and digested for use by the body,
dietary fiber remains reasonably intact during its trip
through the factory. Vegetables, fruits, nuts, seeds,
beans, and whole grains all contain high levels of dietary fiber.

### *DIETARY FIBRE – A KEY TO HEALTH*

Dietary fiber can be classified as either *soluble* or *insoluble*. The soluble kind dissolves into a gel-like material, which can help to regulate blood glucose levels,
thus lightening the load for the pancreas and its production and delivery of insulin. It can also help to

lower cholesterol. Soluble fiber can be found in oats, beans, barley, apples, and citrus fruits. Insoluble fiber remains intact throughout digestion, and facilitates the movement of materials through the digestive factory. Examples of insoluble fiber are nuts, beans, and vegetables, such as cauliflower and potatoes. *Resistant starch* functions much like soluble fiber, wherein it travels relatively intact through the factory until it finally meets up with the good bacteria in the colon. Friendly gut bacteria outnumber the body's cells by a staggering ratio of ten to one. Resistant starches and fibers, including bananas (slightly under-ripe), grains, seeds, and legumes, feed these bacteria. The digestion of these materials by the bacteria causes fermentation, which results in by-products that reduce inflammation and help to improve insulin sensitivity. This means that your body can maintain a healthy relationship with insulin, rather than constantly provoking its release. Insulin can effectively perform its function, rather than being overproduced and over-released into the bloodstream, thus causing the body to eventually build up a resistance to its effectiveness. Insulin resistance has been linked to several serious diseases, including metabolic syndrome, Type-2 diabetes, obesity, heart disease, and Alzheimer's disease. Dietary fiber and resistant starch are essential dietary elements in the prevention of disease through nutrition.

A whole food plant based diet will ensure that you are eating naturally occurring dietary fiber from nuts and seeds, beans, vegetables, and fruits. By eating those foods in their natural form, you will get the full benefits of their components. Precooked and processed foods, such as flours, crackers, and chips, lose their essential benefits through these means of preparation. It is important to remember the word "whole" in whole food plant based nutrition. As for fruit, it is important to eat the fruit rather than to simply drink the fruit juice. Fruits are high in naturally occurring fructose, or sugar. They are also high in dietary fiber. By reducing the fruit to juice, however, the fiber is lost and all that remains is the sugar. Even though this sugar still comes from a fruit, it is still sugar, and is treated that way by your body. Eating the fruit intact, however, will allow the naturally occurring fiber to slow the absorption of the fructose thus preventing a sudden rush of liquid sugar. Nature provides us with its own prepackaged snacks in the form of fruit. They are all unique with different tastes, and they contain the exact amounts of the nutrients that they are meant to be providing. Juicing, even cold-pressed, is a form of processing the fruit, and should be avoided. Eat the fruit as a fruit and reap the full benefits of its components: fructose, vitamins, minerals, fiber, and antioxidants. You will feel full after the consumption of fruit, whereas juice, which may even be an addition to a meal, will not give you a feeling of satiety, regardless of containing the same number of calories. While these sugars are not necessarily refined, the body will receive them in the same way that it might receive the sugar from drinking a bottle of soda. Naturally occurring dietary fiber should be a regular part of your diet, and it is readily available through whole food plant based food choices.

## *ANTIOXIDANTS VS. FREE RADICALS*

*Free radicals* and *antioxidants* are interactive examples of action and reaction. Free radicals are atoms that are generated by the foods that we eat, the medicines that we take, the air that we breathe, and the water that we drink.

These substances can include fried foods, alcohol, tobacco smoke, pesticides, and air pollutants. Basically, oxygen in the body splits into single atoms with unpaired electrons. Electrons like to be in pairs, so these atoms, called free radicals, scavenge the body to seek out other electrons so that they can become a pair. This process, however, causes damage to cells, proteins, and eventually DNA. Antioxidants, on the other hand, neutralize the free radicals. Antioxidants are molecules in the cells that prevent free radicals from scavenging the electrons in the body and thus causing damage. They can sacrifice an electron to bind with the free radical without compromising their own structure, thus neutralizing the free radical without causing any harm to the body. Although the body produces some antioxidants in-house, the majority of these compounds are obtained through nutrition. Examples of foods that contain a high level of antioxidants are berries, tomatoes, broccoli, spinach, nuts, and green tea. Some of the specific antioxidant compounds include *beta-carotene*, and other *carotenoids, lycopene, lutein, resveratrol*, vitamins C and E, and other *phytonutrients*, the nutrients found in plants.

Free radicals are not, however, completely negative. Intense aerobic exercise, such as running, can cause a chain of chemical reactions that allows free radicals to be formed at a faster rate. These free radicals are thought to help reinforce the immune system, which builds strength by managing this type of naturally occurring situation. Free radicals can be beneficial in small amounts. They prompt your cells to become stronger over time by increasing your body's ability to produce antioxidants. Free radicals also serve as important signalling molecules for numerous functions in your body, so eliminating of them entirely could prove to be counterproductive.

Antioxidants are the "defenders" that help to offset free radicals, "the destroyers." The aggression from harmful environmental substances, or those ingested by an individual due to less than optimal lifestyle choices, will need to receive some sort of defence so as to avoid damage to the cells of the body. We can reduce the intake of known sources of the scavenging free radicals, just as we can increase the consumption of antioxidants in order to reduce or neutralise these attacks. Ideally, it is beneficial to do both.

Antioxidants can essentially be found in whole plant foods, including fruits, vegetables, whole grains, nuts, seeds, legumes, and certain herbs and spices. It is necessary to include a wide range of these foods so as to avoid the progressive destruction and premature aging of cells, proteins, and the precious DNA that defines who we are. Remember that telomeres are the sheaths that protect the DNA within our cells. Unchecked free radicals in the body are destructive to telomeres, shortening them and making them more vulnerable to damage. Nutritional and lifestyle choices help to ensure the longevity of the body's cells, which, in turn, help to protect us from illness, premature aging, and disease.

## CHAPTER NINE

*Damage and Prevention*

C ell damage generally results in disease. When these foundational components of the body begin to break down, malfunction, or mutate, the results are often dramatic. The human body is an incredibly resilient and complex organism. It is also inherently fragile and in constant effort to seek and maintain its healthiest balance. When we offer the best input to our factory, then the operation and output are generally smooth and efficient. Inversely, when we provide our bodies with foods that are fried or processed, are difficult to digest, are high in fats, sugars, and oils, or if we pursue lifestyle habits that expose the body to detrimental input, such as alcohol, tobacco, and other detrimental substances, then we are opening a door for disease and grave malfunction to enter the factory grounds and disrupt its operation. Environmental stress factors already stack the deck against us. Noise, air quality, jobs, living conditions, and myriad other factors of daily life trigger the hormonal machine of the endocrine system to keep churning in an effort to keep us balanced. We can find strategies to lower the impact of these stress triggers, but they may still have a profound effect on us. Food, however, is completely with our realm of control. If we can eliminate poor food choices as negative impact factors to our overall health, then we are preserving our bodies, and relieving them of the arduous task of dealing with accumulated detrimental input. The cells of our bodies can only do so much. Our endocrine system can only do so much.

## CELLULAR DAMAGE – DESTROYING THE FOUNDATION

Damage can occur to our cells in the forms of chronic *inflammation*, *oxidative stress*, and *insulin resistance*. The foods we eat can either increase inflammation, or prevent it. Our unhealthy food choices can literally feed our imbalances and create considerable health issues. Inflammation is part of the body's immune response. It triggers a chain reaction that begins with the release of white blood cells to the site of the inflammation in order to solve the problem. There are two types of inflammation: acute and chronic. Acute inflammation is a localized, precise, and short-term issue that needs attention from the immune system, such as a cut on leg or a sore throat. Immune cells are called in for reinforcement and deal with the problem at hand. Swelling, heat, and pain are all parts of the healing process. As the body's immune cells do their jobs, the body heals, and the inflammation subsides. Chronic inflammation, on the other hand, can have long-term, pervasive effects on the whole body. This type of systemic inflammation can be a primary contributor to the development of disease.

## *INFLAMMATION*

Chronic, low-grade *inflammation* does not have symptoms. It can be triggered by perceived internal threats without a specific malfunction or injury to heal. Serving as the army of our internal defenses, white blood cells are enlisted into action in the event of chronic inflammation, and spread throughout the body, with no distinct location and no clearly defined task. Eventually, they act to fulfill their destiny as white blood cells, and start to attack the healthy tissues and cells of our internal organs. The foods that we eat can become the enemy for which these white blood cells are waiting. Perhaps, the enemy could appear from *leaky gut* syndrome, in which indigestible food can create small perforations in the lining of the small intestine, allowing substances like bacteria, toxins, and undigested food to leak into the bloodstream where it does not belong. After all, food that is being digested is meant to remain in the intestine, and not to be floating around in our blood. Our immune system recognizes these escaped food particles as foreign invaders, and attacks them. As leaky gut syndrome continues, so do the foreign invaders, and so does the response from the immune system, and so on. The result is persistent, chronic inflammation throughout the body. Foods that promote inflammation in the gut are refined carbohydrates and sugars due to the fast release of glucose into your bloodstream after consumption. This rapid spike in blood glucose levels can cause an increase in *cytokines*, the messengers of inflammation. Alcohol is another source of inflammation for our cells, destroying our telomeres and exposing our DNA to damage. Anti-inflammatory foods include nuts, flaxseeds, and leafy green vegetables, all of which contain Omega 3's. This compound helps to keep our cell structures intact. Our cells can also convert Omega 3's into hormones that help to regulate inflammation. *(Blackburn and Epel).*

## OXIDATIVE STRESS

*Oxidative stress* comes from an unfortunate, positive ratio of free radicals to antioxidants. When the damaging free radicals outnumber the healing antioxidant compounds, oxidative stress can occur. Oxidation in the world around us is often referred to as rust. The cells in our bodies essentially undergo a similar, damaging process in the presence of unchecked free radicals. Oxidative stress specifically damages the lipids, proteins, and DNA of our cells, causing them to age prematurely or even resulting in complete system failure for those cells. The presence of ongoing oxidative stress within our bodies can eventually lead to major diseases, including arteriosclerosis, cancer, diabetes, rheumatoid arthritis, stroke, and other cardiovascular diseases. As we saw in the previous chapter, free radicals can come from the foods that we eat, the water that we drink, the air that we breathe. As we can truly be impactful with regard to our food choices, it is important to avoid high glycemic foods that are rich in refined carbohydrates and sugars, all forms of processed meat and red meat, cooking fats and oils, fried foods, and alcohol. Foods that combat these free radicals with high levels of antioxidants include whole cereals, beans, green tea, herbs and spices, and generous daily portions of fruits and vegetables, especially berries, leafy greens, artichokes, and cruciferous vegetables, like broccoli, cauliflower, and cabbage.

## INSULIN RESISTANCE

*Insulin resistance* is yet another physical condition that can arise in our bodies due to repeated and continued detrimental food choices. High intake of refined sugars has been linked to insulin resistance. Refined sugars from sweets, juice, sodas and the like enter the bloodstream without the benefit of dietary fiber to slow them down. This rapid increase in blood glucose (sugar) levels prompts the pancreas to produce and release insulin into the bloodstream. The continuous striving for balance is underway. Insulin triggers responses in certain cells that allow them to absorb the glucose from the bloodstream to use as energy, thus returning the sugar levels in the blood to a normal state of balance. Sounds easy. As a general rule, it is easy. When excessive amounts of sugar are dumped into the bloodstream all at once, however, this system is put under pressure. Perhaps not all of the sugar that is present in the blood can find an outlet. If this is the case, the pancreas continues to recognize the blood glucose levels as elevated, and continues to produce and release insulin to reestablish balance, and the cycle continues. This is one reason why it is a better choice to eat a fruit, which has its natural fiber to help with digestion and a slower release of its sugars, than it is to drink a fruit juice, which no longer has the fiber of the fruit, yet has maintained its full sugar content. Sugar is a highly addictive substance, and overconsumption is common. To avoid unwanted sugar intake, read labels, and look for words like *sucrose*, *glucose*, *fructose*, *maltodextrin*, and *high fructose corn syrup (HFCS)*, amongst others.

Animal products also play a huge role in this dark film of insulin resistance. A saturated fatty acid, known as *palmitate*, is found in animal products, including meats, processed meats, dairy products, and eggs, and has been linked to insulin resistance. Intake of the saturated fats from animal products can become toxic, which causes inflammation and oxidative stress in human adipose (fat) tissue. This leads to an impairment of *mitochondrial* (cell) function and insulin signaling, resulting in insulin resistance. It is as if the insulin, striving to achieve balance by facilitating the passage of blood glucose into the cells, continues to knock on the cell's door without ever getting a response. The cell never even hears the insulin knocking. Blood glucose levels thus remain high, and insulin production and release continues in a response to the high sugar levels in the blood. This can develop into a continuing cycle, during which the body gradually builds up a resistance to the excessive insulin and becomes unaffected by its presence.

Insulin resistance is known to lead to a higher risk of developing cardiovascular disease and Type-2 diabetes, as well as various forms of cancer, including bladder, breast, colon, cervix, pancreas, prostrate, and uterus. Obesity is a condition that promotes the development of insulin resistance. Foods that create favorable conditions for the onset of insulin resistance are animal products, such as meat, dairy, and eggs, and heavily processed versions of food, including grains, sugars, and cooking oils. This condition can be avoided or improved by eating healthy plant-based fats, which are found in nuts, seeds, avocados, and olives, as well as previously mentioned anti-inflammatory foods, such as vegetables and herbs and spices. Foods that are rich in anti-inflammatory properties and antioxidant compounds will help to alleviate and avoid chronic inflammation and oxidative stress. These potentially ongoing states within the body are hugely detrimental to overall health, and are also inherently linked to the dangerous condition of insulin resistance.

The cells of our body need us to look after them. They are reactive units. What we put into our bodies directly affects the functioning of these primary components. Cells collectively make up every tissue in the human body. If we nurture them and protect them, they will thrive. If we neglect their wellbeing, and allow damaging compounds to attack them, they will inevitably suffer and malfunction. Once again, it is a good idea to take a step back to look at the whole person. We are affected by our environments, our families, our personalities, our jobs, and certainly by the foods with which we choose to nourish our bodies. We can influence our health at every moment of the day with the lifestyle choices that we make, and, most certainly, with the choice of the food that goes to ensuring the proper functioning of the factory. This is perhaps the most crucial lifestyle choice of them all.

### NATURE DEFENDS AGAINST STRESS

One of the foundations of Ayurveda is balance. The philosophy and practice of Ayurvedic medicine is centered on the maintenance and reestablishment of balance. Imbalance, mental, emotional, or physical, is thought to be the origin of disease. Our physical body functions much in the same way. The endocrine system is constantly striving to maintain balance within the organs and systems of our bodies. Each endocrine gland excretes the hormones for which it responsible in an effort to maintain and reestablish homeostasis within the constantly changing entity that is the human body. Ayurveda is simply an alternative medical philosophy and practice that strives to assist our bodies in this eternal pursuit of balance. Life Knowledge. The more we understand about our whole selves and take into account the parameters that are beyond our control, the more we will be able to act positively upon the parameters that are within our realm of influence. Thus begins the prevention of imbalance (disease) and the healing of the whole person. When we begin to implement proactive and positive behaviors toward ourselves, the influence of these actions can spread from the narrow domain of acting upon that which is within our control to impacting what was at one time beyond our jurisdiction.

Imagine that you have a domineering and dismissive colleague at work. This person's main line of communication is sarcasm. Nothing that you do is ever good enough, and open discussion with this person is not part of the existing dynamic. You may go to work feeling defensive, powerless, or detached. These emotions may provoke stress responses in your body from the moment you wake up in the morning. Feelings of dread may creep into your consciousness, affecting not only your work life, but your family life and your personal health as well. Of course, the foods that you eat can help to offset the damage that may be inflicted to your physical being; however, no healthy diet is going to change the behavior of this person who weighs heavily on all aspects of your life. You must accept that that person will not alter his or her way of being. The only remaining option is to either quit your job, or change the way that you receive the energy that this person throws your way. Perhaps a simple, or not so simple, reframing of the situation in your own mind will suffice to make you feel better, or perhaps you will opt for some form of meditation to help you reposition your emotional responses with regard to this person. Whichever strategy you employ, the end desire is the same: to neutralize negative input so that you are no longer damaged by it. This is adaptation. It is what has allowed our species and all others to endure over time. Those who are able to adapt are the healthiest, and the healthiest of any species are the ones who survive. Perhaps, your repositioning, or adaptation of yourself, with regard to this sarcastic colleague may eventually even alter his or her way of being toward you.

## *ADAPTOGENS – MAINTAIN BALANCE, REDUCE STRESS*

Amazingly, nature provides us with numerous compounds whose jobs it is to adapt, and to help us to adapt as well. These unique plants and herbs are appropriately known as *adaptogens*. These naturally occurring substances offer support to the adrenal system, which oversees stress responses, or the *fight or flight r*eactions with which we are regularly faced. These compounds help to balance hormones in an effort to deal with stress on a daily basis. They adapt to what your body needs, and they have the ability to assist your body in regulating itself to increase or decrease hormonal levels depending on specific needs as they arise. Their jobs are, once again, all about balance and the prevention of negative impact on the human organism. Adaptogens are essentially herbs, and some mushrooms, that contain high concentrations of antioxidants, anti-inflammatory substances, and phytonutrients that add to their impressive list of benefits. These substances are not considered by Western medicine to be actual medicines, as they are not synthetically produced and tested in a pharmaceutical facility. It would be impossible to analyze adaptogens in the reductive, isolated way that has become customary in conventional medical research. Adaptogens are complex, bilateral compounds, which means that they can stimulate the function of under-producing organs, or even whole body systems, or, inversely, they can calm the functioning of overactive organs and systems, and perform these opposing tasks all at the same time. These are healing compounds as much as they are preventative ones, stimulating substances as much as calming ones. Their effects will thus vary from person to person, due to their adaptive nature. Unlike prescription, pharmaceutical drugs, which contain isolated compounds, adaptogens contain several, co-existing compounds that enhance one another and work together to perform their tasks.

The mainstream health community does not currently officially recognize benefits of adaptogens. Conventional medical research on the isolated substances within one adaptogenic plant would be reductive and perhaps inconclusive, as it is the complex, interactive nature of these plants and herbs that make them so unique and effective. If individuals could begin to prevent potential health threats and treat existing imbalances with plants and herbs, then conventional health professionals and pharmaceutical industries could potentially be slightly less in demand. Current and past practitioners in the oldest existing health care system in the world, Ayurveda, frequently employ adaptogens to prevent disease and to reestablish healthy balance within the bodies and minds of their patients. The objective is personal empowerment and naturally occurring, non-synthetic remedies are tools.

Adaptogens with known health benefits to the human body include:

*Ashwaganda* – Ashwaganda is an antioxidant that supports the cardiovascular, endocrine, immune, and nervous systems. It can help to promote sleep and improve physical recovery.

*Astragalus* – Astragalus has antibacterial, antiviral,

and anti-inflammatory properties. It supports and strengthens the immune system.

***Bacopa*** – Bacopa can help to regulate cortisol levels during stress reactions. It can also improve cognitive performance.

***Bilberry*** – Bilberry can be effective in the prevention and treatment of urinary tract problems.

***Cinnamon (Ceylon)*** – Cinnamon has strong antioxidant and anti-inflammatory properties. It lowers blood sugar levels, and improves insulin sensitivity, thus working as an effective anti-diabetic substance. Cinnamon may help with neurodegenerative diseases, such as Parkinson's or Alzheimer's, and help to protect against cancer. It also has antifungal and antibacterial properties.

***Cordyceps*** - Cordyceps is a medicinal mushroom that is known to effectively enhance immune function.

***Dang Shen*** – Also known as codonopsis, dang shen helps to defend against extreme stress, anxiety, trauma, and fatigue.

***Elderberry*** – Elderberry can help to reduce fever and support the immune system.

***Eleuthero*** – Also known as Siberian Ginseng, eleuthero helps to strengthen the immune system, and improves stamina and endurance.

*Ginger* – Ginger has a broad spectrum of health bene-fits. It offers immune support, relieves nausea, aids in digestion, and is an effective anti-inflammatory.

*Ginseng* – Ginseng can work to prevent cancer, fa-tigue, and inflammation, and can be helpful in the treatment of existing cancer and diabetes. Can be re-ferred to as Panax, or Asian Ginseng.

*Green Tea / Matcha* – Green tea contains high levels of antioxidants (*catechin & ECGg*), which are highly effective in preventing & fighting cancer. Contains the amino acid *L-Theanine*, which enhances the produc-tion of dopamine & serotonin, which help to increase memory and concentration, as well as increasing en-ergy levels & endurance. Also, contains Vitamins A and C, potassium, calcium, iron, and protein.

*Guduchi* – Guduchi is a detoxifying, rejuvenating, im-mune-boosting adaptogen. It is known to be effect-ive in numerous disorders, and can help mitigate the negative effects of chemotherapy.

*He Shou Wu* – This Chinese herb is known for its neuroprotective properties, and helps in the treat-ment of blood, kidney, and liver disorders.

*Holy Basil / Tulsi* – Holy Basil is anti-inflammatory and antimicrobial. It can reinforce the circulatory, immune, and nervous systems, and can be effective in cancer treatment. Holy basil also helps to the body to stabilize the stress hormone cortisol. Tulsi means "the incomparable one."

***Jiaogulan*** – This herb is known to reduce LDL cholesterol, stabilize blood sugar, and improve immunity.

***Licorice Root*** – Licorice root supports immune function. It protects the thymus from being damaged by cortisol. Licorice root can affect blood pressure, so should be used under medical supervision only.

***Lycium / Wolfberry / Goji Berry*** – This adaptogen contains *flavanoids*, which are antioxidant and anti-inflammatory *carotenoids*. It supports liver and kidney function, and can be used to help strengthen weak muscles and ligaments.

***Maca Root*** – Also known as Peruvian Ginseng, maca is known to increase strength, stamina, and libido.

***Neem*** – Commonly referred to as "the village pharmacy," neem is known to neutralize free radicals, and can be used in the treatment of numerous ailments and diseases.

***Nutmeg*** – Nutmeg can be effective in the treatment of digestive disorders.

***Reishi*** – Reishi mushrooms can help in the treatment of fatigue, respiratory issues, cancer, liver problems, and heart disease.

***Rhodiola*** – Rhodolia can be used to treat a wide variety of symptoms. It helps to restore and stabilize blood glucose levels, and can support fertility. It also increases alertness, fights depression, and lessens fatigue.

*Shatavari* – This herb is thought to support fertility in women.

*Trikatu* – Trikatu strengthens the upper GI tract, and enhance digestive function and the absorption of nutrients.

*Triphala* – This adaptogen regulates, strengthens, and tones the digestive system. It is detoxifying and anti-inflammatory to the lower GI tract, and can help with sluggish digestion and bloating. Triphala is complimentary to trikatu.

*Turmeric* – Also known by the name of its active ingredient, *curcumin*, this adaptogen enhances flexibility and reduces inflammation. It can be used in cancer treatment due to its properties as a growth inhibitor for tumors.

While some of these adaptogens may seem exotic and foreign to some people, and are currently labeled as tools of "alternative medicine" by conventional health professionals, they have been used for centuries as effective methods for treatment in Chinese medicine and Ayurveda. Others, however, are more familiar and readily available in most grocery stores and markets, such as cinnamon, turmeric, ginger, and green tea. By including these in your daily food regime, you can give your body a natural boost that can keep conventional medicine and synthetic pharmaceuticals at bay.

As we have seen, stress factors can be external or internal, beyond our control or within our control. The body does not necessarily differentiate, and certainly does not care from where the stress originates. It receives the stress as a threat to the body's precious equilibrium, and simply deals with it by using the tools that are at its disposal. These tools are generally in the form of hormones, which are in constant states of adjustment to create balance. The body's capacity for adaptability is remarkable. It is our responsibility to our personal factory to do whatever is possible to keep it running smoothly. We can reduce incoming stress by choosing foods that promote health, rather than opting for foods that are known to promote disease. Our body systems, organs, and hormones cannot be asked to work their regular shift plus double overtime shifts. They already work around the clock, 24/7. Creating additional work simply overloads the system, which will inevitably experience difficulties and breakdowns in the form of preventable diseases. By including adaptogenic plants and herbs as an integral and regular part of our healthy nutritional intake, we can lend an extra helping hand to our bodies by creating a reduced and easier workload. The organs that produce the crucial hormones that keep us in balance will get encouragement to function properly. Their health will improve. Your health will improve.

## CHAPTER TEN

*A Brief History, Part IV*

In 2011, I was involved in a high speed, hit and run motorcycle crash. I was riding on a major highway when a speeding car drifted across lanes and hit my back wheel, sending me on a slide across three lanes of traffic until I finally came to rest in the emergency lane on the side of the road. Luckily, the cars behind me had seen the incident unfolding and slowed, some even stopped. The driver of the speeding car spun a few times and finally came to a stop down the road, before fleeing the scene. Apparently, the driver was texting before he made impact with my motorcycle. The results of that incident could have been dramatic. My protective gear did its job, my skin was undamaged, and my other injuries were certainly more contained than they could have been. I ended up with fractures to my left elbow and my right scapula. My right patella was shattered into six pieces. I spend a few days in the hospital to undergo surgery to repair my knee, which was wired and pinned. I was placed in a hip-to-ankle cast, which I would wear for six weeks. My body had been structurally damaged, but nothing was remotely life threatening. I knew, however, that it would be a long road to recovery.

As I lay in the hospital bed awaiting my surgery, I was already researching what I could to do ensure that my body would repair itself to the fullest. I made a list of foods to avoid and foods to choose. My obscure habits from my college days of randomly maintaining food journals suddenly came rushing back. I remember smiling to myself and thinking that, regardless of what path we walk, there is a certain continuity that is inherent to each of us. During the six weeks that my leg was completely immobilized, I followed a strict, self-imposed nutritional regime. I wanted to avoid gaining weight due to my lack of mobility, and also wanted to give my body the necessary tools to heal itself. I asked the surgeon about this, and he just smiled and vaguely reassured me that nothing in my life should change. His dismissiveness of my questions on nutrition told me that I was onto something.

After the first week, I was able to get myself around without the help of crutches, and walked as best I could as often as I could for as far as I could. This was in November in a cold, rainy country. My motivation for recovery was high. I returned to gym workouts so as to keep my upper body strength relatively intact. Once the cast was to be removed, I wanted to be ready to go. At the end of the six weeks, I began physical therapy on my knee. Due to the length of immobility, I could no longer bend my leg. My muscles had atrophied, my tendons and ligaments had stiffened, and scar tissue had formed like glue around the injury. This period was extremely painful and difficult. I recognized the gravity of the full extent of the structural damage of my injury at this point. I continued with my disciplined and perhaps extreme nutritional regimen. The first physical therapists told me that I would be lucky to recover a knee bend of 90 degrees. This was devastating to me. I was an avid and frequent cyclist and runner. According to this restrictive prognosis, I would not be able to do either of those things. The doctors and physical therapists comforted me by reminding me that it could have been worse, and that I should feel fortunate. They would consider 90-degree mobility as a complete success. It was difficult for me to accept this, so I did not. I persevered with my healing diet, and sought out more specialized recuperative therapy.

I finally landed upon a wonderful sports injury therapist, who vaguely concurred with my dietary choices, but who reassured me that I could expect recovery, which would allow me to return to most of my past activities with the possible exception of running. My job at the time required me to be highly mobile and relied heavily on leg strength. I spent most of my working days at cycling races, marathons, and triathlons standing on the back on a motorcycle with a camera on my shoulder. My injuries had kept me out of work for nine months. After a year, I was able to get my leg around the full rotation of a pedal stroke on a bicycle. Four years after my accident, almost to the day, I began to run again. The first physical therapists and doctors had underestimated the capacity for recovery. I was stubborn and did not want to accept their expectations as absolute truth. I have now regained knee joint mobility in excess of 135 degrees, nearly equivalent of my healthy knee.

I attribute my recovery to a certain personal stubbornness, to physical perseverance, to some dedicated sports therapists, and also to the effects of my obscure dietary modifications. Perhaps the effect of these nutritional choices is mere coincidence; however, the result of having surpassed my recovery expectations speaks for itself. Conventional medical professionals might say that it is difficult to know with certainty just how much of my physical recuperation was or is due to diet, and how much is due to other factors. No advice on my dietary habits was made or offered during the entire recovery process. Perhaps, a holistic approach would have been a worthwhile alternative. I decided to undertake that on my own, and I now enjoy a level of recovery that is nearly without limitations. I did what was in my power to help my damaged tissues repair themselves and regain normal function. I preferred and still prefer to stack the deck in my favor rather than to ignore potential paths of prevention and recovery.

## CHAPTER ELEVEN

*Foods to Choose, Foods to Avoid*

The healing properties of certain foods are undeniable, as is the destructive nature of others. We have looked at the preventative and curative properties of adaptogen plants and herbs. Certain foods, known as *superfoods*, carry these same attributes, but as complete food items.

## SUPERFOODS – PREVENTION OVER CURE

*The Meriam-Webster Dictionary* defines *superfood* as "a food (such as salmon, broccoli or blueberries) that is rich in compounds (antioxidants, fiber, or fatty acids) considered beneficial to a person's health." While this definition is a colloquial one, there is no true scientific or medical definition of a superfood. Much like adaptogens, superfoods do not contain one isolated compound that has one isolated effect on the human organism. These foods contain multiple compounds with multiple positive effects on the body. These are foods that must be viewed from a broad, whole perspective. Superfoods contain high levels of vitamins and minerals, and are natural sources of antioxidants, which shield our bodies from cell damage, inflammation, and help prevent disease. These foods are generally low in calories and high in nutrients, making them nutrient dense foods. These foods contain compounds that assist the human organism, rather than stress factors that complicate the body's functions. Superfoods are the nutritional equivalents to adaptogenic plants and herbs.

Superfoods include the following:

**Açai** - This superfood is rich in antioxidants (*anthocyanins*), which help fight cancer and heart disease. Açai also contains oleic acid

**Avocados** - This fruit contains Vitamins K, C, B6, E, *folate*, and high amounts of potassium. They also contain fats that increase *HDL cholesterol* (the good kind) and reduce *triglycerides* (dangerous fats). They help to stabilise blood sugar, and reduce the risk of prostate cancer, and, generally, have low pesticide levels.

**Beetroot** - Beetroot contains high levels of antioxidants, Vitamins A & C, which help to fortify the immune system and reduce risks of cancer and other degenerative diseases. Beetroot also contains potassium and fibre for proper functioning of vital organs and the digestive system, as well as high levels of Vitamin B9 (folate), which ensures proper nerve structure and function, and reduces the risk of dementia.

**Blueberries** - These berries are high in fibre, vitamins C & K, and *manganese*. They boast the highest antioxidant concentration of any fruits, which helps to prevent or reduce risk of cancer, urinary tract infections, high blood pressure, diabetes, and DNA damage. They help to maintain muscle integrity after strenuous exercise.

**Broccoli** - This cruciferous vegetable contains high levels of carotenoids, and *sulforaphanes*, which help to flush cancer-causing elements from the body. Broccoli reduces tumour growth, and increases digestive health due to high fibre content. Broccoli contains protein.

**Chia Seeds** - These tiny seeds are high in Omega-3 fatty acids, fibre, and protein. They also contain antioxidants, calcium, and magnesium.

**Chlorella** - Chlorella contains high levels of protein, Vitamin C, and iron, as well a variety of minerals, and a wide range of anti-oxidants, Omega-3 fatty acids, and fibre. Chlorella can help with cholesterol levels, immune system function, blood sugar regulation, aerobic endurance, and blood pressure stabilisation. Chlorella is usually consumed in a powdered form, either mixed with other foods or water.

**Cacao Powder** (**raw or non-alkalized**) - Cacao contains flavonoids, which are known to lower blood pressure and improve blood flow to the brain and the heart.

*Goji Berries* - These berries are rich in antioxidants, and contain high levels of Vitamin C, which boosts the immune system and fights cancer. They are also known to stabilise blood sugar levels and detoxify the liver.

*Hemp Seeds* - These hulled seeds are high in protein and contain all essential amino acids needed for growth and repair. They also contain significant levels of magnesium and potassium.

*Nutritional Yeast* - This is a good source of protein and fibre. It is often fortified with Vitamin B12, which is essential for normal brain and nervous system function.

*Papaya* **(organic only)** - This tropical fruit contains vitamins C and E, *beta-carotene*, and *lycopene*, which help prevent heart disease and improve digestion. It is important to consume only organic papaya. Pesticides used in it's farming are numerous and easily absorbed by the fruit.

*Pineapple* - This fruit is high in dietary fibre and Vitamin C. It helps to increase immune function, lower *LDL cholesterol* levels, and reduce free radicals in the body. It can also reduce the frequency of bronchitis, sore throat, and gout.

*Pomegranate* - The seeds of this fruit contain Vitamins A, C, E, K, and folic acid, and high levels of antioxidants, which can reduce heart problems, prevent cancer (prostrate & breast) & *osteoarthritis*, and help to control diabetes. They also contain high levels of potassium and fibre.

**Spinach** - Spinach contains Vitamins A, K, D, and E, calcium, as well as many trace minerals. It also contains Omega 3 fatty acids, and a multitude of antioxidants, which help to prevent inflammation and disease. Spinach has a highly alkalising effect on the body (counteracts an acidic state). It has also been shown that there is a chemical reaction that occurs when chewing leafy greens that activates anti-inflammatory substances.

**Seaweed** - Seaweed provides high concentrations of Omega-3 fatty acids, which defend against sudden heart attack and stroke. Seaweed also contains many important minerals (calcium, magnesium, iron, potassium, iodine, & zinc).

**Spirulina** - This algae is a good source of protein, copper, and iron, as well as Vitamins B1, B2, & B3. It offers high antioxidant and anti-inflammatory properties, can lower LDL cholesterol and triglyceride levels, and can also be used to treat allergic rhinitis. It is usually consumed in a powdered form, and added to other foods.

*FOODS TO AVOID FOR DAMAGE CONTROL*

By choosing to nourish the cells of our bodies with the highest quality nutrients, we take crucial steps toward prolonged and sustained health. Whole food plant based choices, with an array of superfoods, coupled with adaptogenic plants and herbs will bolster your body systems and help them to function at their highest levels. Your cells will be receiving the nutrients that they need to operate in a stress-free environment. Body weight will be optimal and stable, thus steering us away from myriad preventable diseases. The performance and output of your personal factory will be at its highest level. When we offer food to our bodies that inhibits proper functioning, however, we create an environment that is favourable to the formation of disease. Our cells require nutrients, not calories, to maintain healthy activity. If our food choices are low in nutrient density and dietary fibre, yet high in saturated fats, our bodies will suffer. In other words, if food intake is relatively devoid of positive nutrition, our cells will be crying out for nutrients, regardless of how many calories have just been dumped into the factory.

Many highly marketed and commonplace food items can cause grave damage to the body. Food industries and their marketing campaigns do not necessarily have the health of the consumer as a primary concern. Profit is the main pursuit, as it is logically with most companies. Saturated fats, salt, and sugar tend to be highly addictive food elements. These items are often added to packaged, processed foods, simply to create cravings and food addictions, and to promote overconsumption and overeating. More foods sold to us, translates as higher profits for the company. Industrial farming and agriculture exist to provide the highest amount of sellable food to the largest number of people. As a result, even some "natural" food choices are rife with potential disease-creating ingredients.

The following foods and food groups are known to promote disease and to diminish the quality of human health.

## WHEAT AND WHEAT BY-PRODUCTS

**Gluten** - Whole wheat contains a substance called *gluten,* which, as its name implies, has a glue-like aspect. Basically, gluten contains proteins that are inflammatory to the digestive system and create an immune response. Our immune system flags these proteins as foreign invaders and attacks in efforts to eradicate them for the benefit of our health. The internal walls of the intestine are attacked as well, however, as the gluten has a tendency to stick to these tissues. Approximately 1% of people have a true allergy to gluten, known as celiac disease, which can be a serious immune disorder with sharp, dangerous symptoms. A much larger percentage of people are thought to be gluten sensitive, which means that they will have some symptoms, like pain, anaemia, bloating, and tiredness when ingesting gluten. Gluten is also though to increase permeability of the intestine, resulting in *"leaky gut,"* which is known for triggering its own set of symptoms and immune responses. Gluten has been associated with a variety of brain disorders, including *cerebellar ataxia* (motor disturbances caused by brain lesions), *schizophrenia, autism*, and *epilepsy*. On the slightly less dramatic end of that spectrum, a feeling of confusion, or *"brain fog"* can result from the consumption of gluten. Gluten may also cause addictive responses in the brain. Some of the proteins in gluten get broken down during digestion into *opioid peptides*, which signal an addictive response in the brain, thus potentially creating food cravings.

***Phytic Acid*** - Wheat contains *phytic acid*, which binds with certain minerals, including calcium, zinc, and iron, and inhibits their absorption during digestion. Calcium reduces acidity (*pH*) levels in the body. When ingested calcium is bound to phytic acid, which prevents its absorption, acidity levels can rise. Our parathyroid glands sense these changes in acidity, and send hormonal messages requiring the body to pull calcium from the bones in order to balance the *pH* levels. Calcium is one of the primary mineral components of bones, so the result of this process is that bones can become more frail and brittle.

## *ANIMAL DAIRY PRODUCTS (MILKS – CHEESES - YOGURTS)*

Human breast milk is the perfect nourishment for the development of a baby human. Similarly, cow's milk is the perfect growth formula for baby cows. Human consumption of animal milk is known to promote major diseases. It is naturally high in saturated fats, which contribute to heart disease, stroke, diabetes, high cholesterol, and obesity.

*Lactose Intolerance* - Dairy products contain a naturally occurring sugar, known as *lactose*. In humans, an enzyme called *lactase* is responsible and necessary for the breakdown of lactose for proper digestion. This is particularly important in infants, who need lactase to digest breast milk. As children grow older, however, lactase production is greatly diminished. 75% of adults no longer produce enough lactase to correctly digest the lactose that is present in all dairy products. These people would be considered as lactose intolerant. Symptoms of lactose intolerant individuals usually arise between thirty minutes to two hours after consumption. These can include stomach pain, gas, and bloating, as well as diarrhea and constipation.

*Milk Allergy* - Milk allergy, on the other hand, is a true food allergy, and is the most common allergy amongst young children. Symptoms arise due to an allergic reaction to a protein in milk, and can also include stomach pain, nausea, and diarrhea, as well as respiratory difficulties, swelling, and skin rash. Consumption of dairy products can lead to compromised digestion and discomfort, which affects every aspect of the digestive process, and will hinder the proper breakdown of foods as well as their healthy absorption.

*Ingested toxins* - Dairy cows, especially in industrial-scale situations, may live in less than optimal sanitary conditions. Antibiotics are used on a large scale to mitigate the spread of disease. Growth hormones and oestrogen are administered in order to maintain the cows in a state of permanent lactation. Pesticides and chemical fertilisers are used to produce high amounts of feed that are required for dairy cows. As toxins are stored in fat cells, these ingested products inevitably become part of the milk that is then extracted for sale and consumption. As these cows are permanently producing milk and having this milk extracted mechanically, there is a high probability and frequency of *mastitis*, or udder infection. Pus is discharged from these infected udders and also makes its way into the milk.

While the dairy industry builds its sales and public awareness campaigns to advertise dairy products as health promoting and high sources of calcium, there is no evidence to support these claims. There are, however, established links between dairy consumption and heart disease, prostate cancer, and osteoporosis.

## *SUGAR*

Refined sugar is perhaps the most damaging substance for the human body. Sugar is responsible for chronic and pervasive inflammation and increased levels of LDL cholesterol. It has toxic effects for most systems, organs, and tissues of the holistic body, including the following: brain, mood, teeth and gums, joints, skin, heart, liver, pancreas, kidneys, body weight, and sexual health.

*Body Weight* - Refined sugars are empty calories. The more sugar you eat, the more weight you will gain. Obesity is a grave condition that promotes numerous other functional health problems.

*Brain* - Sugar is a highly addictive substance, due to the chemical releases that it triggers in the brain, which in turn trigger cravings and addictive response patterns.

*Heart* - Excess sugar in the bloodstream leads to high blood pressure, which can eventually lead to insulin resistance, Type-2 diabetes, cardiovascular disease, and stroke.

*Joints* - Generalised inflammation due to sugar intake can also create and worsen soreness in the joints, can increase the risk of developing *rheumatoid arthritis*.

*Kidneys* – As the kidneys are the filter system for the body's fluids, they suffer tremendously under diabetic conditions. Kidney function can also be compromised due to obesity, which is a primary side effect of consuming empty calories, including refined sugar.

*Liver* - The liver is a key organ in the processing and storage of sugar. An overload of sugar will cause the liver to become insulin resistant, which translates to the fact that the liver will no longer be affected by the hormone that controls blood glucose levels. The result can be Type-2 diabetes.

*Mood* - Spikes and crashes in blood glucose levels due to sugar intake can lead to feelings of euphoria and anxiety.

*Pancreas* - The pancreas is the creator and provider of insulin. When the body gradually becomes resistant to the effects of this hormone, the pancreas keeps producing it in an effort to make some impact on blood sugar levels. The pancreas will eventually become overworked and will experience dysfunction. The result is Type-2 diabetes.

*Sexual Health* - As sugar consumption affects blood flow, erectile dysfunction can occur.

*Skin* - Premature aging of the skin is another side effect of the chronic inflammation that accompanies sugar intake.

***Teeth and Gums*** - Sugar promotes tooth decay and gum disease. This chronic disease creates an on-going inflammatory response, which can be a precursor to heart disease.

Sugar is gratuitously added to most packaged foods in order to "enhance flavour," so many hidden sugars are lurking in foods where we would never expect to find them. Again, it is necessary to read labels in order to avoid falling into the dangerous cycle of insidious food cravings and addictions, as well as the negative spiral of uncontrollable weight gain.

Look for any of the following ingredients as sugars:

*Glucose*
*Fructose*
*Maltodextrin*
*Sucrose*
*High Fructose Corn Syrup (HFCS)*

High Fructose Corn Syrup is a highly refined and processed sweetener that is found in a vast amount of packaged and processed foods. HFCS can increase LDL cholesterol levels, which can lead to Type-2 diabetes. This artificial sweetener is extremely high in calories, and can cause damaging weight gain more rapidly than any other food ingredient.

## ARTIFICIAL COLOURINGS

Food dyes and artificial food colourings are generally made from petroleum, which also serves as source for gasoline, diesel fuel, asphalt, and tar. These dangerous chemical additives can be found in soda drinks, sports drinks, baked goods, processed meats, candies, and desserts, and are added for the sole purpose of making these products more visually appealing. Many negative side effects have been linked to food colouring and food dyes. These include:

*Cancer*
*Chromosomal damage*
*Brain tumours*
*Thyroid tumours*
*Bladder tumours*
*Lymphomas*
*Hyperactivity and ADHD*
*Neurochemical and behavioural disorders*
*Allergies*
*Eczema*
*Insomnia*
*Aggression and violent behaviour*

A small handful of these compounds have been banned in a minority of European countries, while only one has been excluded for use in the United States; most food dyes, however, continue to be added to processed food products around the world. They are recognisable in ingredient lists, as they are denoted with a capital letter E, or FD&C. Natural food colourings come from various plants and food compounds, including turmeric and paprika.

## *ARTIFICIAL SWEETENERS*

Artificial sweeteners are prevalent throughout the westernised countries, and can be found in most sweet tasting packaged food products, and nearly all diet soda drinks. These chemical compounds offer a sweet taste without the high calorie content of sugar. Once these chemicals head into the factory for digestion and absorption, however, they are broken down into highly toxic chemical agents. These can wreak havoc in the body, damaging tissues, organs and entire body systems. These compounds generally start off as sugar, and undergo a chemically altering process that subsequently renders them calorie free although highly toxic. The side effects of these compounds can have devastating effects on the human organism.

*Aspartame* – aka *Equal* and *Nutrisweet*. This compound is 200 times sweeter than sugar. It is composed of *phenylalanine, aspartic acid, and methanol.* Phenylalanine has been linked to depression, and emotional and psychotic disorders. Aspartic acid has a stimulant effect on neurons and contributes to the destruction of cells. Methanol is a *neurotoxin*, and its absorption in the body is increased when heated to over 30 degrees Celsius (86 Fahrenheit). Average human body temperature is 37 degrees Celsius (98.6 Fahrenheit). When surpassing this heat threshold, methanol breaks down to *formaldehyde*, a highly *carcinogenic* compound that damages the nervous system. Associated health risks are memory loss, oxidative stress to the brain, headaches, mood disorders, and dizziness. Aspartame can also adversely affect the liver and kidneys.

***Sucralose*** – aka *Splenda*. This sweetener is 600 times sweeter than sugar. It is essentially sugar that has been transformed by adding three *chlorine* atoms to its chemical structure. *Chlorinated sucrose* was originally discovered in research toward the development of new insecticide compounds. It was not intended for consumption. Chlorine is a highly effective antiseptic, which, when ingested, damages healthy gut flora (bacteria), which increases the frequency of *candida*, *irritable bowel syndrome (IBS)*, and *colitis*, amongst others. Sucralose has also been shown to damage the thymus gland, and increase inflammation in the kidneys and liver.

***Sodium Benzoate*** – This substance is used as a preservative, and is used in soda drinks, sports drinks, and processed foods. Sodium benzoate is a water-soluble preservative salt, which has been associated with neurodevelopmental disorders, such as *ADHD*, as well as *asthma*. This substance is commonly mixed with vitamin C in soda drinks and energy drinks. The combination of these two compounds creates *benzene*, which is highly carcinogenic and linked the onset of leukemia and lymphoma.

***Acesulfame K*** – aka *Ace, Ace K, Sunette, Sweet One,* and *Sweet'N Safe.* This is a potassium salt that contains *methylene chloride,* and is present in sugar-free chewing gum, candies, sweetened yogurts, and alcoholic beverages. This compound cannot be broken down by the body is has been linked with metabolic disorders.

***Saccharin*** – this artificial sweetener is prevalent in many non-prescription and children's medications, including cough syrup. Possible side effects of saccharin include nausea and digestive issues, and its consumption has been linked to bladder cancer, amongst others.

***Xylitol*** – aka *Erythritol, Maltitol, Mannitol,* and *Sorbitol.* These alcohol sugar derivatives can be found in sugar-free gum, mints, candies, and frozen desserts, and can cause bloating, gas, cramping, and diarrhea.

These compounds are highly potent artificial sweetening agents, which can lead to insulin resistance via food addiction. The sweeter the food, the more the body is going to crave that sweetness. Thus begins a domino effect of food cravings for low nutrition foods, leading to overeating of those foods, leading to extra empty calories, leading to obesity, leading to insulin resistance, leading to disease. Although these artificial sweeteners may contain no calories, they do carry potentially devastating negative side effects, and the foods with which they are associated are generally low in nutrients and high in calories and processed ingredients. Recommended natural sweeteners would be maple syrup, stevia, and dates.

## ARTIFICIAL FLAVOUR ENHANCERS AND PRESERVATIVES

Artificial flavours are made from a combination of chemicals that are found in inedible ingredients such as paper pulp or petroleum. They are created to replicate the exact taste and smell of their naturally occurring counterparts.

*Monosodium Glutamate* – aka *MSG*. This flavour enhancer is regularly added to processed meats, canned soups and vegetables, and Chinese food. It first originated from combining *gluten isolate* with *sulfuric acid*. The United States Food and Drug Administration (FDA) places MSG on their list of foods that are "generally recognised as safe" (GRAS); however, some symptoms have been reported after the consumption of foods that contain MSG. These symptoms can include, dizziness, headaches, allergies, and nausea, amongst others.

*Nitrites* and *Nitrates* – These preservatives are commonly found in processed meats, lunch meats, and cured meats. They help to retain consistency in colour over long periods of time. They can contribute to high blood pressure, and have been associated with an increased risk of oesophageal, stomach, and colon cancers.

**Potassium Bromate** – This compound is used in bromated flour, which is used in processed breads, even those labelled as whole grain and "healthy." This additive has been linked to thyroid disease, DNA damage, and kidney problems.

**Butylated Hydroxyanisole** – aka *BHA*. This additive is commonly found in chips and preserved meats, and has been linked to fertility issues in women.

**Butylated Hydroxytoluene** – aka *BHT*. BHA and BHT are close cousins, as both are added to foods as preservatives. BHT can be found in cereals and sauces, as well as in dry, processed baked good, including crackers and cookies.

**Propyl Gallate** – This preservative is often used in conjunction with BHA and BHT. Propyl Gallate is found in foods that contain edible fats, such as vegetable oil, sausage, processed meat, and some cereal products. Its function is to keep the fats in those foods from becoming rancid over time. Propyl Gallate can also be found in some shampoos and cosmetic products as a means to preserve their colour. It has been associated with the onset of allergic reactions, including asthma and skin irritations. Liver and kidneys are also thought to suffer in the presence of Propyl Gallate, and the risk of certain cancers may also increase.

***Propyl Paraben*** – This additive can be found in processed baked goods, such as muffins. It is a harmful chemical that negatively affects testosterone levels in men, and fertility in both men and women.

All of the aforementioned substances have been deemed "*generally recognised as safe*" by the United States Food and Drug Administration. These additives and preservatives are readily used in highly processed and commercially packaged food items. Their presence in these items is undeniable. With the existence of recognisable physical symptoms from the consumption of these chemicals, it is wise to read food labels, and to make proactive, informed choices as to whether or not you want to put them into your body. These chemical additives have been approved for public consumption and widespread use in processed food items; however, they still remain chemicals that are not naturally occurring and/or destined for the human organism. The body will naturally struggle to break down and absorb foreign chemicals and their by-products. This may create stress for numerous organs, and the chemicals themselves may have varying adverse effects from person to person. As we have seen, the body continuously strives for balance. The presence of harmful chemicals as food items in the body will generate added stress and will certainly create imbalance. By avoiding foods with these types of additives, we are lightening the body's workload and safeguarding the organs that must process these chemicals. Even if there is a lingering doubt as to whether or not something might be destructive to your health, perhaps it's a wise decision to eliminate it. The "generally regarded as safe" label for foods from the FDA is almost as reassuring as a mechanic who tells you that the brakes on your car will probably work most of the time.

## FISH AND SEAFOOD

While concentrated levels of healthy Omega 3's can be found in some fish, mercury is a dangerous substance that finds also its way into the waters of our oceans and streams, and therefore into the fish that live there. Pollution from plastics also has tremendous residual effects on fish and seafood.

*Mercury* and *Methylmercury* – Mercury is a by-product of fossil fuel combustion and waste incineration. When this compound is in contact with bacteria, it becomes *methylmercury*, which is a poisonous substance. An article entitled "Can Eating Fish Be Dangerous? The Facts About Methylmercury," published by the National Center for Health Research states with regard to methylmercury, "Unfortunately, this toxin is in the fish we eat. Methylmercury can accumulate in streams and oceans. It also accumulates in the food chain, as each fish absorbs all the mercury of the smaller fish or organisms it has eaten. That is why the oldest and largest fish, such as shark or swordfish, have the highest levels. Methylmercury levels are higher in people who regularly eat fish." Methylmercury is a neurotoxin, meaning that it toxin for brain tissues and functions. The risks associated with this poisonous substance can include depression, blurred vision, and impaired hearing and speech in adults, while infant exposure can lead to difficulties with attention span, language development, visual-spatial skills, memory, and coordination. *(Diana Zuckerman, PhD, Anne Gallo, MS, Madeleine Levin, MPH, Celeste Chen, and Michela Leboffe Tabaku, National Center for Health Research).*

*Plastics* – Pollution levels due to plastic in the oceans is a huge problem for all levels of marine life. Plastics are not biodegradable; however, they are in a continuous state of fragmentation. *Microplastics*, or small particles of disintegrated plastic, pollute the waters in which they are present. These plastics include *nylon, polystyrene (Styrofoam)*, and *polyethylene*. It is thought that plastic can serve as a means of transport for toxic substances such as organic pollutants and heavy metals. When fish or seafood filter the water in which they live, some of these plastic particles remain in their organism, and are subsequently ingested by humans who eat the fish or seafood.

**MEAT – ALL VARIETIES**

The consumption of meat is a leading precursor to a wide array of potential and preventable health risks. Animal protein has been widely advertised as healthy and necessary for the human diet due to its high protein content. It is true that animal flesh contains a complete array of amino acids, those important building blocks of proteins, which allow our bodies to function. Animal flesh also contains high levels of saturated fat. Animal flesh is the only dietary source of cholesterol. Animal flesh contains no dietary fibre. Consumption of fat and cholesterol, and inadequate fibre intake have all been linked to the onset of a vast number of major diseases.

*Cancer* – *The Cambridge English Dictionary* defines *carcinogen* as "a substance that causes cancer." The *International Agency for Research on Cancer* classifies carcinogenic groups of food products. Their classification system sets Group 1 carcinogens as definite causes of cancer, Group 2 as probable causes of cancer, Group 3 as possible causes of cancer, while Groups 4 and 5 are exempt as causes of cancer. Processed meats are considered a Group 1 carcinogen, along with items including, arsenic and asbestos, air pollution, alcohol, and all forms of tobacco smoke. Pork, beef, and lamb are classified as Group 2 carcinogens, along with malaria, coal tar, and insecticides.

The *World Health Organisation* has stated that consumption of processed meat increases the risks of colorectal cancer by eighteen per cent. A 2014 Harvard study found that just one serving a day of red meat during adolescence was associated with a twenty-two percent higher risk of pre-menopausal breast cancer. The same red meat consumption in adulthood was associated with a thirteen per cent higher risk of breast cancer overall. During the processing or cooking of meat, carcinogenic substances called *heterocyclic amines* are formed from the inherent presence of amino acids, sugars, and *creatine* in the meat. This chemical transformation occurs in all forms of red meat as well as in chicken. The hormones that are present in meat have also been linked to increased risk of cancer. Meat also contains *Insulin-like Growth Factor 1 (IGF-1)*, which is a *peptide* that stimulates cell growth. High levels of IGF-1 have been linked to greater risk of breast and prostate cancers.

***Heart Disease*** - Animal products (meat, dairy, and eggs) contain cholesterol and saturated fat. Extensive scientific research has linked dietary cholesterol to cardiovascular disease. In the United States alone, over 2,000 people die every day from some form of preventable cardiovascular disease. Saturated fat is present in all animal products, including fish, chicken, and turkey (even when cooked without the skin). High LDL cholesterol levels can leave streaky deposits of fat on the interior walls of your arteries. These fat deposits accumulate and thicken, thus complicating and compromising blood flow. If the heart does not get enough oxygenated blood, the result is a heart attack. Decreased blood flow to the brain can result in a stroke. High sodium levels in processed meats can lead to high blood pressure. Approximately thirty per cent of annual deaths in the United States can be attributed to preventable heart disease. Six in ten preventable heart deaths occurred in people under the age of 65. The World Health Organization has found that "cardiovascular disease (CVD) causes more than half the deaths across the European Region," and that "eighty per cent of premature heart disease and stroke is preventable." High cholesterol and high blood pressure are known precursors of cardiovascular disease.

*Diabetes* - Insulin resistance is the primary warning light prior to hitting the wall of the disease known as Type-2 diabetes. As we saw in Chapter XX, consumption of the saturated fats found in animal products creates insulin resistance due to the inflammation and oxidative stress that the fatty acid palmitate initiates in the adipose tissue. Nitrates found in processed meats can cause high blood pressure, which creates favourable conditions for the onset of insulin resistance, followed by a diabetic condition. Consumption of processed meats is associated with a nineteen per cent higher risk of developing Type-2 diabetes. During a recent study in Israel, "researchers gathered information on meat-eating habits from 357 adults, ages 40 to 70 years. They divided them into those who ate less than 1.1 daily portion of meat - that was the median intake - and those who usually had more. A portion was considered about 3.5 ounces (100 grams) ... Out of the total participants, 39% had liver disease and 30% had insulin resistance."*(Does Eating Red Meat, Processed Deli Products Boost Your Diabetes Risk? by Kathleen Doheny and Elena A. Christofides MD, FACE. Study leader: Shira Zelber-Sagi, RD, PhD).*

**Inflammation** - Stress that is caused to the multitude of body systems and organs due to meat consumption can create favourable conditions for chronic inflammation. The body's reaction to perceived threats, and real functional threats, is low-grade chronic inflammation. *Methionine*, an amino acid found in high levels in meat (pork, beef, and lamb), has been found to increase inflammation.

**Body Weight** - Due to the high level of saturated fat intake that is inherent to meat consumption, maintaining healthy body weight as a meat eater can be challenging. It is thought that meat may contribute to obesity to the same extent as sugar. University of Adelaide Professor Maciej Henneberg puts it this way: "Whether we like it or not, fats and carbohydrates in modern diets are supplying enough energy to meet our daily needs. Because meat protein is digested later than fats and carbohydrates, this makes the energy we receive from protein a surplus, which is then converted and stored as fat in the human body."

**Food poisoning and toxins** – Rachel Krantz writes, "The U.S. Department of Agriculture (USDA) reports that seventy per cent of food poisoning is caused by contaminated animal flesh. Foodborne diseases, such as E. Coli, Salmonella, and Campylobacter, cause an estimated 76 million illnesses, 325,000 hospitalizations, and 5,000 deaths in the United States each year. Eating meat puts you at a greater risk for food poisoning because animal products are often tainted with fecal contamination during slaughter or processing." Unwanted compounds, including antibiotics, administered growth hormones, and synthetic steroids are also likely to be present in meat products, and can be toxic for hormone-balancing endocrine system and the filtration and conversion organs, the liver and kidneys. Toxins are stored in fat cells, and, as we now know, meat contains high levels of saturated fats.

*Dietary Fibre* – Dietary fibre is an essential element of the health of our gastrointestinal tract. It is responsible for keeping things moving through the length of our digestive factory, and helps with the absorption of nutrients. Meat contains no dietary fibre whatsoever. It is thus more difficult to digest, and can be destructive to the all-important healthy bacteria that reside within our intestine and ensure the health and proper functioning of our immune system. Whole grains, nuts and seeds, and vegetables generally take twelve hours to digest, keeping the factory clean and moving. Meat, on the other hand, may take up to seventy-two hours to fully digest, overworking the factory and making it seem more like an employee sit-in rather than an efficient as-sembly-line.

The consumption of meat carries a high amount of inherent danger. Given that adequate protein is avail-able from whole grains, nuts and seeds, and vege-tables, the benefits of eating meat would not appear to be worth the risk of confirmed, chronic, and poten-tially deadly diseases.

## CHAPTER TWELVE

*A Brief History, Part V*

November 2013, I attended my first yoga class. I was initially reluctant due to the injuries I had sustained from my motorcycle accident. Although my body had recovered more completely than anticipated over the past two years, there remained pain and some mobility limitations. I had convinced myself that these would prevent me from participating in a yoga practice. I was wrong. I discovered a new way of perceiving my physical body as well as the very solitary joy of a meditative practice. A sixty-five minute yoga practice somehow reintroduced me to the familiar gratification of the keeping food journals, reading philosophy, and riding my bicycle for hours and hours.

I began reading books that I had not thought about for many years. Words and ideas from these books had become part of who I was, like some sort of genetic modification of the soul. I had not consciously understood this until I dove into writings that seemed profoundly and intimately familiar to me. Ideas that had formed who I was as an adult were now being reabsorbed by the adult that they had helped me become.

Convoluted, perhaps, yet ultimately exhilarating. My mind discovered a new sense of ease that it had not experienced in many years. I devoured these books, and deeply enjoyed the feelings that they provoked within me. Everything that I had learned before came flooding back to me. Ideas regained their proper place in my consciousness. The dots were connected. My random choice to abandon eating animal products thirty years ago no longer felt so random. I questioned how I could have gone back to eating animal products. I experienced clarity. Meditation practice that I had respected in my daily routine at that time had evolved over the years into a sort of moving meditation that I naturally fell into while running or cycling. Reconnecting with the philosophical writings and thoughts that had shaped my lifestyle allowed me to consciously recognize that they had been with me all along. It was like reconnecting with an old friend.

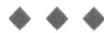

The summer of 2013 saw some drastic changes in my father's declining health. He had undergone his ileostomy intervention. The doctors advised him to follow with a brief treatment of chemotherapy just to eradicate any remnants of the cancer that seemed to find new hiding places in his body. He was physically weak and compromised. Whatever the doctors recommended, my father abided. The first chemotherapy session had dramatic negative effects on him. His body nearly threw in the towel completely, and his mind would be altered for the remainder of his life. This engaging, intelligent man had been transformed into a distant, intellectually detached shell of his former self, who now found it almost beyond his powers to hold a meaningful conversation.

We knew that the end of his life was quickly approaching. He, however, was white knuckled, trying to cling to a life that was rapidly slipping through his fingers. I organized my work in Europe so that I could be at home with my parents in the States for the two months before Christmas. This was sure to be my father's swan song. We were all in agreement. There would be no more medical interventions, no more dramatic lifesaving attempts. We simply made sure that he was maintaining his schedule of IV hydration that had become necessary for his physical comfort. Nothing more. My father's tenacity, however, proved to be unyielding. He survived those months, and beyond.

During this time of relative family cohesion, I continued to read and attend yoga classes. I began to enjoy the physical practice more and more, as I could feel my body adjusting to this new activity. My mind was thriving as well. Everything became purposeful. Knowing that I would remain with my family for a few months, I had brought my bicycle. I would get up early in the morning, and go out for a ride before any-one was awake. This was my meditation, and it made more sense now than ever before. After a couple of hours and a few dozen miles, I would return to my parents' house to start the day with them. Some days, an early yoga class would replace the bike ride, and, other days, the class would be in the evening. During the afternoons, I would stay with my father mostly, offering my mother a break from her caretaker duties, and sometimes taking my father out on a randomly conceived field trip, just to change things up for him.

I wanted to know more about my father. I tried talking with him about his own father, his past, his feelings. These were the things that defined my father, and I had not previously known about them. Nor, as it turned out, had I known much about him. I had con-structed an image of my father according to my ex-periences, and now I wanted to understand what had made him the man that he was. The secrets that my father kept locked up so tightly during his entire life were destined to remain within him. He would never utter a word about his feelings. They were would re-main only in the shadows of his own being. I knew not of his memories, nor of the emotions that accompan-ied them, but I could finally see a demeanour in my father that I had never seen before. His eyes held sad-ness and panic.

My father would resist a few more close brushes with death before he would finally capitulate some months later. Somehow, he had held the missing piece that would complete my puzzle, and that piece only materialised after his death. I felt empowered and whole. Everything mattered. Everything had consequences.

These weeks would prove to be pivotal for me. I was starting to put together some crucial pieces of my life – my job, my family, my physical being, my thoughts, and my actions as a whole. I had always viewed these as separate elements. I recognized a certain pinball tendency in myself, much like my father. Flow with the river. The various aspects of my life took on a new dimension when I began to see them as the whole of me.

I continued to practice yoga, and to get lost in the obscurity of my philosophy books; however, these were no longer separate things. I understood that the physical practice of yoga was intimately enmeshed with its philosophy and its history. It was a lifestyle. It was not just a strenuous workout, or relaxation therapy. There were ethical practices that had been associated with the physical practice of yoga for centuries, and this connection resonated deeply with me. It was familiar. I had always had the pieces; I just never saw how they fit in with each other. My father's passing brought it all together. The unity of the pieces now made perfect sense to me.

◆ ◆ ◆

Correct physical alignment is one of the principles of yoga. This helps to avoid physical injury, and to offer stimulation and targeted work to the muscles, joints, and organs that are supposed to be receiving that attention. Alignment is a necessary and disciplined part of a yoga practice. I had always understood this as strictly physical. Alignment, however, goes far beyond the body. It includes all aspects of existence. The discipline of physical alignment in postures, while necessary for the health of the body, is also the outward manifestation of the alignment that must be practiced within. Moral and ethical alignment with actions defines the individual, as well as considerations for the physical body. Actions are the outward expressions of inward intentions, and coherence of these aspects of the self leads to balance. Holistic integrity. Holistic balance. Much like the endocrine system perpetually balances our internal factory, actions regulate and balance us with the outside world. The physical practice of yoga strengthens the body and the mind, and demonstrates the truth that proper alignment will inevitably increase balance, everywhere. It all made perfect sense to me. Finally.

*Yogic Philosophy*

"The restraint of the modifications of the mind-stuff – this is Yoga." Sri Swami Satchidananda's translation of the Sutras from their original Sanskrit thus defines yoga. In other words, tuning out the chatter that rattles endlessly through the mind.

The *Yoga Sutras of Patanjali* is the foundational text on the practice of yoga and yoga philosophy. These writings are generally thought to have originated around 300 CE, and are divided into four separate chapters, or books. Essentially, the Sutras offer practical insight into leading a purposeful and meaningful life in the quest for higher understanding and enlightenment. Modern yoga is founded upon the philosophy and practices that are presented in these writings.

### EIGHT LIMBS OF YOGA

The *Eight Limbs of Yoga*, as outlined in the Sutras, offers a comprehensive, holistic approach to human existence. They encompass ethical actions and observances. They address the physical body, as well as the emotional, psychological, and the spiritual being. The Eight Limbs offers an evolving roadmap of the constant striving toward right living and the eventual attainment of enlightenment. All aspects of the individual are considered. They exist simultaneously and build upon one another.

Limb One, *Yamas*, and Limb Two, *Niyamas*, deal with actions and emotions. These are the foundations. As individuals, the actions in which we engage tend to define who we are. No hiding. No excuses. Our entire being is influenced, shaped, and eventually defined by what we do. Our actions are the results of our choices. We are continuously confronted with choices, which determine our actions, which, in turn, determine the next choices and actions, and so on. The Human Condition. We can influence the path upon which we walk at any moment in our lives. Adjustments, rectifications, and changes are perpetual. A holistic view of the self is essential. We are not pieces of a whole. We are the whole.

### YAMAS AND NIYAMAS

Yamas are five moral restraints. These ethical prescriptions are aimed at helping the individual to elevate himself from his lower nature. These are actions and behaviours that affect others and the self. Upholding these restraints amounts to maintaining an ethically elevated way of life. Niyamas are five observances. These address attitudes, thoughts, and beliefs, and are meant to cultivate positive qualities that, in turn, encourage a favourable environment for healthy living, spiritual enlightenment, and a liberated state of existence. The Niyamas can serve as the internal structure for upholding the Yamas. Respecting the Yamas and the Niyamas is entirely down to personal choice, discipline, and conviction. Adherence to these principles of behaviour and thought helps to keep us on track.

We have seen that minimised stress and maximised balance can make the difference between health and disease. The food choices that we make are fundamental to this process. Actions that are fully within our realm of choice are limited. We have communication. No one can force an individual to use or not use certain words or means to communicate ideas. Those are purely individual. Education, culture, and emotion can create parameters for communication, but how one actually chooses to communicate is strictly a personal choice. The physical actions that we execute with our bodies are also under our absolute control, barring a compromised physical or medical condition. We can choose to raise our hand in a classroom if we have a question to ask. We choose to accelerate or slow down a car that we are driving. No one can do it for us. We are in control of those actions. The primary action that keeps everything going, however, is eating. Without the fuel that we choose to put into our bodies, it would be pointless, and physically impossible, to consider these questions. Food intake is one of the primary choices that an individual can make. Life literally depends on it. Choices start every time that we receive that ghrelin signal telling us it's time to feed the factory. Our mind starts to rifle through the options. What am I hungry for? What flavour is my body asking for? What is available? What should I eat? What do I really want to eat? The questions are endless. Once we have sifted through the possibilities and narrowed things down to where we have decided upon what we are going to put into our mouths, we proceed to action. All of these responses are within each person, are different for each person, and will vary over time. Some deciding factors may be emotionally driven, while others may be intellectually motivated. These decisions all result in an individual choice. That ultimate gesture of putting hand to mouth to feed the factory is purely personal.

If the reduction of stress and the creation of balance for optimal health are important to you on a personal level, then discipline will be capital if you are to achieve these goals. Discipline is inherent in the concept of restraint. What you put into you body does matter. Remember, we are holistic beings. We are the whole, not just a collection of parts. The body and the mind are so intricately intertwined that it is impossible to separate physical processes from emotional and mental wellbeing. It is fundamental to maintain a disciplined approach to one of the only elements of life that we actually control on a consistent level. Our actions are of the utmost importance; the thought process behind those actions is equally significant. This discipline with regard to food affects not only our personal, physical health, but can have far reaching ethical implications as well. When we violate basic moral principles, we either do so voluntarily through an absence of consideration, or we do so due to ignorance. Both can be overcome. The moral restraints of the Yamas create parameters that serve as reminders within our endless unfolding of choices, and steer us in the direction of controlling personal desire in exchange for the creation of slightly more elevated states of being.

### AHIMSA

*Ahimsa* refers to non-violence. It literally means non-harming, and intimates the pursuit of compassionate behaviour toward all sentient beings. This refers to all creatures that can suffer and feel pain. Ahimsa has direct and obvious applications toward food. Do not kill or cause suffering to animals. Do not slaughter them to eat their flesh. Ahimsa is one of the easiest Yamas to recognise in a yogic lifestyle, which predicates a diet that does not include animal products. We could walk away from the notion of ahimsa at this point, and its connection to nutrition would be adequate; however, it actually goes much deeper. The concept of non-harming also includes speech, thoughts, and actions directed inward, as well as actions directed toward other beings. As we have seen throughout the previous chapters, consumption of animal products is a major contributor in the promotion of major disease. Harm is clearly done to the animals through slaughter and industrial livestock farming. Harm is also done to ourselves when we eat these foods. Physical damage eventually ensues from animal products. If we look at a broader scale of life interactions, there is room to think that damage is also being done on a more universal, spiritual level. When we consume animal products, we are nourishing ourselves with the dead flesh of another being, and the pain and suffering that accompanies this surely cannot be a good thing to absorb into the cells of our bodies. The concept of non-harming can also be applied on a broader, global level. Livestock farming has a tremendous environmental footprint. It directly contributes to land and water degradation, acid rain, compromised biodiversity, deforestation, and coral reef degradation. Livestock farming is the largest contributor to negative climate change. By choosing against animal consumption, we can also take a small step toward reducing the harm that is being done to our environment and our planet. Ahimsa also includes thoughts. It can be as simple as looking in the mirror with an approving pair of eyes, seeing and accepting the whole, imperfect person without negative judgement. When we begin to approach all aspects of our lives through the filter of ahimsa, the effects spread like wildfire. Buddha is credited with the following statement: "The thought manifests as the word; the word manifests as the deed; the deed develops into habit; and habit hardens into character. So watch the thought and its ways with care, and let it spring from love born out of concern for all beings... As the shadow follows the body, as we think, so we become."

### *SATYA*

*Satya* is truth. Authenticity and truthfulness in words, thoughts, and deeds are the foundational concepts of satya. When we live in accordance with our beliefs, this is a form of truth. When we thoughtfully express our opinions and convictions, this, too, is truth. Satya should not override or conflict with ahimsa. Speaking our truth in such a way that it is disrespectful or condescending to others would thus be inappropriate and destructive. Satya can be applied to food by recognising the truth about certain food items. Being truthful with yourself as to the knowledge that eating a bowl of broccoli is a healthier choice than eating a slice of pizza, regardless of which one you desire or choose. Satya is not lying to yourself with regard to the risk of certain health issues that are related to the consumption of certain foods. Satya is being responsible for those things that are within our realm of control, such as food choices and eating habits. Satya is going to a restaurant with friends who all order meals that do not correspond with your own food choices, and still ordering a meal that is in alignment with your own lifestyle. Truth about foods that can damage you body is sometimes difficult to hear and sometimes difficult to ignore. Truth can be a predominant factor in your decisions, internally and externally, every time you sit down for a meal or grab a snack.

## ASTEYA

*Asteya* is non-stealing. Clearly, this means not taking something that belongs to someone else. This can refer to possessions, thoughts, experiences, and well-being. Asteya is seated in the realm of self-confidence. If you trust in what you have as being what you need, then there is no motivation to "steal" something that you don't have. Asteya can thus apply to cravings; that drive to have something that you do not have, the feeling that something is missing. Avoid foods that promote cravings, such as sugar, salt, and fried foods. Asteya can also apply to overeating, which can spring from the desire to simply fill a void, physical or emotional. Asteya would be to not use food as compensation. On a more physiological level, we have seen that certain foods and their components can steal other compounds from the body. Phytic Acid in wheat "steals" iron, zinc, and calcium from other nutrients and prevents their absorption. Higher acidity levels in the body, caused by certain foods, can signal the parathyroid glands to leach or "steal" calcium from the bones to re-establish balance in the body. As far as food is concerned, asteya could involve choosing not to consume foods that are known to steal nutrients from the body, or force the body to "rob Peter to pay Paul," as we have seen with calcium redistribution. Generosity is also inherent to asteya. Giving is a greater action than taking. Offer your body the finest nutrients possible, and avoid taking away from your own factory by pushing it toward system failure. Be generous with your health.

## BRAHMACHARYA

*Brahmacharya* comes from the root words *Brahman*, meaning "universal consciousness," and *charya*, "to follow." The main principles of Brahmacharya are "right use of energy," and "moderation in all things." It is often reduced in its meaning to chastity or celibacy, which makes it rather unpopular. This is a reductive and only partially correct. Brahmacharya promotes the right use of energy, which implies not being promiscuous if you are single, as this would create energy that is dispersed, rather than focused, and supports fidelity in a committed relationship, which encourages this focus. Brahmacharya is essentially about how and where we direct our energy, and encourages that we strive to move away from external desires, and more toward inward recognition, peace, and happiness. This involves moderation and a certain control of our senses. As we look to apply this to our food consumption, we can see where the idea of moderation finds its place. An easy way to apply this moderation is to serve your food in smaller plates, eat more slowly, and use smaller utensils or even chopsticks. These will all help to moderate the amount of food you are eating and the speed at which you are eating it. If we dig a bit deeper and explore the idea of proper use of energy as it applies to food, we could extrapolate that our energy is primarily a by-product of the foods we eat. So, the idea of not wasting our energy would involve not consuming foods that might deplete our physical resources, such as meat due to its toxic effects and the sluggish digestion that it creates, or refined sugar, which causes rapid spikes and crashes in blood sugar levels that drive us from agitation and euphoria to moodiness, impatience, and confusion. Moderation in all things and proper use of energy are the restraints that are meant to help us take a large step on the path of following the universal consciousness.

## APARIGRAHA

*Aparigraha* is the state of non-attachment, non-possessiveness, and non-greediness. This concept addresses your relationship to objects and to other people. In the Bhagavad Gita, one of the foundational ancient yogic texts that predates the Sutras, Krishna states, "Let your concern be with action alone, and never with the fruits of action. Do not let the results of action be your motive, and do not be attached to inaction." Essentially, it's about the journey, not the destination. When we choose to eat healthy, nutritionally dense foods, we are giving ourselves the tools for an improved journey through life regardless of the destination. We are ensuring optimal health, and we are creating new, positive habits. It would be counterproductive to remain attached to old, unhealthy patterns that might be destructive to our physical factory and our general wellbeing. Dissociate emotion, judgement, and past attachment to these habits. Whether our goal is weight loss, improved overall health, or disease reversal, we should avoid looking to the goal line. We cannot control or foresee the future; however, the actions that we take in the present are the cornerstones of what will happen next. Strive for the purest of actions, and let go of the results.

CHAPTER FOURTEEN

*Environment, Sustainability, and Ethics*

A dopting a whole food plant based lifestyle has far reaching impacts on the current and future health of your body. As we have seen through the chapters of this book, the reduction of undo stress on the human organism plays an integral role in the pursuit of optimal health. A holistic approach to the human body allows us to recognize the interconnections and interdependencies of all parts. If we are respectful and nurturing toward our bodies and minds, we can help to avoid a myriad of preventable diseases. That which we put into the factory determines how well the factory functions. This applies to our thoughts and our actions, and certainly to the food with which we nourish ourselves. Preventing and alleviating stress on the system helps to maintain a state of homeostasis that is unique to each of us.

Balance is that primary concern for optimal health. As an individual, we are one entity in part of a whole that currently includes nearly eight billion individuals. If the choices that we make as individuals affect us profoundly as individuals, then these choices and their subsequent actions will certainly impact the entirety of humanity at least in some small way. Change one element in a complex system, and the entire system experiences change. As an increasing number of individuals make fundamental lifestyle changes, the course of actions on a global scale will begin to experience shifts of greater, long-lasting impact. Mahatma Ghandi is quoted as saying, "You must be the change you wish to see in the world." As the world is made up of individuals, change in the world must begin with the individual. While one may think that eating one healthy meal may not positively impact overall health, making every meal a healthy one will not only change the course of events, it can also repair and restore previous damage.

## ENVIRONMENT - URGENT CONSIDERATIONS

The current state of the world's natural resources is critical. Environmental balance and global health are abandoned for the sake of higher profits and the maintenance of destructive, comfortable habits. It is cheaper and easier to drive through a fast food outlet and pay one dollar for a hamburger, which feeds food addictions, creates disease, and is readily available, than it is to seek out fresh vegetables. Choices to encourage environmental protection and sustainability need to be made more readily. As we look at the onslaught of urgent environmental issues, including global warming and pollution, it is important to acknowledge that these are the results of human choices. The earth's ecosystems are much like our body systems; if one is damaged and diseased, it affects all others. If we can alter the course of chronic disease within our bodies by choosing better foods, we can most certainly do the same with regard to the chronic negative impact we are creating on the planet.

The consumption of animal products is one of the primary causes of the increasing degradation and pollution of our environment. Without reversal of this process, the earth's resources are heading toward the proverbial wall at breakneck speed. It is up to us to reverse the increasing forward momentum of this tremendously frightening steamroller of neglect. The extent of the damage caused by the consumption of animal products must be recognised.

It takes 15,000 litres of water to produce 1 kilogram of beef, while it takes 180 litres to produce one kilogram of tomatoes and 250 litres to produce one kilogram of potatoes.

The meat and dairy industry, in the United States alone, are responsible for approximately 55% of annual water use; domestic use accounts for approximately five per cent. One hamburger uses the equivalent of 660 gallons of water, which is equal to two months of showering.

Waste runoff from cattle and other livestock pollutes

groundwater, streams, and rivers. Manure from agricultural farming contains high levels of nitrogen and phosphor. These compounds create increased algae bloom, which depletes the water of oxygen, thus killing the fish and endangering the health of other animals. Water sources can be contaminated by parasites, bacteria, and pathogens, including E coli, Salmonella, Cryptosporidium, and fecal coliform.

Globally, animal farming uses approximately 70% of the planet's accessible freshwater. This is compared to around 20% for industry, and about 10% for domestic use.

In the United States, of the 330 million acres of available agricultural land, 260 million acres are used to produce feed for livestock.

Widespread use of antibiotics to prevent disease in the overcrowded conditions of factory farming facilities has led to the development of antibiotic resistant strains of bacteria. Growth hormones and steroids are also administered to livestock to accelerate maturation.

*Environmental Working Group (EWG)* estimates that 167 million pounds of pesticide and 17 billion pounds of nitrogen fertilizer are used each year, resulting in in a release of greenhouse gas that is 300 times more potent then carbon dioxide. *(Scientific American)*

According to the *National Resources Defence Council,* factory farms, wherein pigs and other livestock are contained in tight quarters, can produce as much sewage waste as a small city; however, there are no septic tanks or sewage systems to treat this waste.

Livestock animals in the United States alone produce an estimated 500 million tons of manure per year.

Waste runoff form factory farming facilities establishes animal agriculture as the primary source of water pollution. This animal waste runoff contains excess antibiotics, hormones and steroids, and chemical residue from ingested pesticides and fertilizers.

Animal agriculture is directly responsible for an estimated eighteen percent of all greenhouse gas emissions.

The Amazon Rainforest is home to ten percent of the world's known biodiversity. 137 animal and insect species are lost every day due to deforestation. Animal agriculture is responsible for over 91% of Amazon Rainforest destruction. *(How Animal Agriculture Affects Our Planet, Haley Hansel).*

Agricultural livestock occupy approximately 30% of ice-free land on earth.

One and a half acres of land can yield 375 pounds (155 kilograms) of meat. That same amount of land could yield 37,000 pounds (15,000 kilograms) of plant-based food. *(Haley Hansel).*

70 billion animals are raised as food every year.

Six million animals are killed for food every hour.

The average American consumes 210 pounds (90 kilograms) of meat per year.


### SUSTAINABILITY

*The Cambridge English Dictionary* defines *sustainability* as "the quality of being able to continue over a period of time." Sustainability can also be thought of as a means of meeting our own current needs without compromising the ability of future generations to meet their own needs. *(What is Sustainability? McGill University, Canada).* Actions toward this end can help to ensure that the earth's natural resources and environmental systems are kept in balance, and that human communities are able to maintain independent and autonomous lifestyles. By choosing to follow a whole food plant based lifestyle, we can reduce the stresses that animal agriculture imposes on natural resources. As in our own bodies, the dominoes of environmental health or destruction do not fall randomly. They are generally lined up in an orderly fashion, and the tipping of one leads to a systematic cascading downfall of others. However, we can step in at any moment. Change in our personal lifestyle choices will directly affect our health and influence the survival of our environment.

## *ETHICS, FACTORY FARMING, AND FOOD LABELS*

Animals are intelligent and complex. They have complete nervous systems. They can feel pain. They can experience suffering. Humans have the ability to reason and to make compassionate choices. It is here that the ethical question of animal consumption reaches its pinnacle. Aside from a common sense of responsibility of not destroying the environment that we require in order to survive, we must consider, as humans, our ethical responsibility of not intentionally causing pain and suffering to other sentient beings. The results of these considerations are our choices, and these choices will vary from person to person. Facts are the same for everyone; how each person decides to react to those facts is purely individual.

## *ANIMAL RIGHTS: ETHICAL CONSIDERATIONS ON CRUELTY*

The concept of ethics is generally understood as an individual viewpoint on a relatively narrow subject that requires an understanding of what is good and what is bad, of where we have moral obligation or duty. Ethics are not absolute. There are systems, or guideposts, such as the Yamas, that strive to offer some clarity and help to define right action with regard to the crucial questions of human existence. Ethics, however, remain individually defined and understood. As for any choice with which we are confronted, knowledge is an essential tool to help us build an opinion, and to subsequently make a responsible choice. Ethics are always relative and dependent upon knowledge and capability.

*Collins English Dictionary* defines *factory farming* as "...a system of farming that involves keeping animals indoors, often with very little space, and giving them special foods so that they grow more quickly or produce more eggs or milk." These "special foods" include hormones and antibiotics, which accelerate growth and prevent disease, which is rampant due to overcrowding and unsanitary conditions. Over 80% of all antibiotics manufactured are used on livestock animals. The *American Society for the Prevention of Cruelty to Animals (ASPCA)* estimates that over 95% of farm animals in the United States are raised on factory farms. A few complementary ethical considerations might accompany the quest for improved personal health and environmental preservation.

**Chickens** – The United States raises and slaughters almost ten times more birds than any other type of animal. 8.5 billion chickens are killed for their meat yearly. 300 million chickens are used in egg production. These are different breeds of chickens, and both have undergone significant genetic modification over recent years in efforts to make them either more productive or to increase and regulate their size. *(ASPCA)*.

*Pigs* – The United States raises 100 million pigs for food every year. Female breeding pigs, or sows, are kept in "gestation crates," and undergo an endless cycle of artificial insemination, gestation, and nursing their young. This cycle continues over several years, until their productivity begins to decline and they are slaughtered for meat. *(ASPCA)*.

*Cattle* – Factory farmed *beef cattle* are raised outside. To rapidly increase their weight, these animals are fed excessively grain-heavy diet that contains high levels of pesticides and chemical fertilisers, and can cause illness, pain, and premature death.

*Dairy cows* are generally kept indoors, and are continuously maintained in a state of pregnancy, as this is the required condition for production of their milk. Unnaturally high milk production leads to mastitis, a bacterial infection of the cow's udder. After a few years of milk production, these dairy cows are slaughtered for meat.

*Veal calves* are separated from their mothers, the dairy cows, at birth. They are often kept in "veal crates," or extremely confined conditions, in an effort restrict their movement to ensure they do not build up muscle. This keeps their flesh tender. They are fed synthetic formula in an effort to keep their flesh pale, as desired by the consumer. *(ASPCA)*.

***Turkeys*** – Approximately 238 million turkeys are bred and slaughtered for food every year in the United States. Selective breeding and genetic selection to meet consumer preferences for breast meat means that the turkeys' bodies have become disproportionate, which prevent them from naturally mating with one another. They are bred on a continuous cycle of artificial insemination. *(ASPCA)*.

Food labels can be deceiving as well. These are qualifications that animal product producers and suppliers may include on their packaging in an attempt to create separation with their competitors, or to cater to the justifications and desires of the consumer.

***All Natural*** – This qualification does not impact animal welfare in any way.

***Free-Range*** – There is no legal definition for use on eggs, pork, beef, or dairy.

***Humanely Raised / Humanely Handled*** – These are undefined and subjective terms without codified standards.

***Hormone Free / No Hormone Added*** – The use of hormones on pigs and poultry is not approved by law, so the term is meaningless on those animal products.

***Cage-Free*** – On eggs, this label means that hens were not raised in battery cages. On poultry meat and meat birds, this is an empty claim, as these animals are rarely raised in cages. They are, however, crowded into large open sheds where overcrowding is inevitable and disease is a constant threat.

***USDA Organic*** – This is a vague label with poorly enforced regulations for animal farming, with no consideration for transport or slaughter.

Whether you choose to adopt a whole food plant based lifestyle to improve your personal health, to reverse the irresponsible trends of global warming, or to advocate animal rights, all will benefit from your choice. The choices that we make affect us on every level of our existence. Foods that we choose to eat will serve to feed our physical bodies and our mental and spiritual beings. What affects our body will affect our mind. We are whole beings. This wholeness extends to how we interact with the outside world, and how our personal choices influence all elements of life around us. It is action and consequence. It is the stone thrown into the stillness of a winter lake, and the ripples that emanate in succession to the farthest shores.

## CHAPTER FIFTEEN

*A Brief History, Part VI*

P hotographs from moon landings and Mars surveys adorned the space around my father's desk. He had been a member of the team that had helped to make these discoveries possible. He had played a part in pushing back the boundaries of what had previously defined human existence. These photographs were his postcards, his souvenirs, along with his memories of those times. Those photos were framed and displayed with pride and wonderment. When I was a young child, I thought that my father had actually been to those places and taken those pictures himself. They were proof to me that another world existed, and that proof was hanging on the wall over my father's desk. As years passed, those same photographs gave my father feelings of melancholy and nostalgia. He never spoke directly of this, but it emanated from every pore of his being. He had been part of something that had changed the world. He had been part of something bigger than himself.

My father always gazed to the stars for inspiration. He turned to the sky in his efforts to understand the human condition and to give some meaning to his own existence. He understood that he was part of something universally larger. He was awed by the creative brilliance of Beethoven, and the intellectual genius of Einstein. The only time that I ever saw my father cry was standing before Monet's *Waterlillies*. This was the essence of life to him. There was greatness in the human race. Perhaps these were the attachments that he felt to his own father.

I realized as an adult that I had been raised with these feelings. These were part of my emotional and intellectual genetic structure. As a child, I was overwhelmed by the enormity of the universe. I would lay awake some nights trying to fathom the notion of endlessness, which solar systems, galaxies, and universes represented. I tried to comprehend the idea that a star in the sky may have died thousands of years ago, but that we were still seeing it because of the enormous distance and the time it took for the light to reach us. That something can be gone yet we are still seeing it and being influenced by it was an abstract notion for me as a young child. As an adult, I now understand how this is possible, yet I still find myself staring at the sky on a clear night, lost in the stars much as my father had been.

My father always looked outside of himself for answers and determining influences in his existence. He trusted doctors and science. He admired great artists. He was moved by beautiful music. My father never turned within for answers. Perhaps if he had done so, he could have influenced his own life with greater aplomb. Perhaps if he had known that he could affect the intricacies of the universe that resided within his own body, he would have taken care of it in a different way. My father, however, saw himself as an infinitely small speck of paint on the great colourful canvas of existence. He never saw himself as the one holding the brush.

As the light of an extinguished star may continue to shine brightly in the night sky, we, too, hold a power that reaches far beyond our immediate realm of existence. We can make an impact on the world in which we live by planting seeds of kindness and responsibility. These actions are within our reach, and will have consequences for generations that are yet to be born. We can influence the state of our own being, also through kindness and responsibility. These actions will affect us immediately. They allow us to stride through this life, and confront the days before us, with a strong, healthy body, and a mind that blooms in the weather of all seasons.

**END**

# GLOSSARY OF TERMS

*Adaptogen* - a nontoxic substance and especially a plant extract that is held to increase the body's ability to resist the damaging effects of stress and promote or restore normal physiological functioning.

*ADHD* - Attention deficit hyperactivity disorder (ADHD) is a chronic condition marked by persistent inattention, hyperactivity, and sometimes impulsivity. ADHD begins in childhood and often lasts into adulthood.

*Adipose Tissue* - Adipose tissue, or fat, is an term for loose connective tissue composed of adipocytes. Its main role is to store energy in the form of fat. It also cushions and insulates the body.

*Adrenal Glands* – The adrenal glands are small-gland located on top of the kidney. The adrenal glands produce hormones that help control heart rate, blood pressure, the way the body uses food, the levels of minerals such as sodium and potassium in the blood, and other functions particularly involved in stress reactions.

*Adrenalin* – Adrenalin is a hormone secreted by the

adrenal glands that increases rates of blood circulation, breathing, and carbohydrate metabolism and prepares muscles for exertion.

*Agni* – Agni is the deity of fire. Agni also refers to the digestive fire that allows for thorough and comfortable digestion of food.

*Ahimsa* - This is the first of the yamas, and refers to non-harming or non-violent behaviour.

*Aldesterone* - The aldosterone hormone is a hormone produced by the adrenal gland. The hormone acts mainly in the functional unit of the kidneys to aid in the conservation of sodium, secretion of potassium, water retention and to stabilize blood pressure. It regulates water and salt balance.

*Alkaline* - Alkaline means that the pH of your body is in a more alkaline rather than acidic state. The body is always trying to maintain equilibrium at a pH of 7.365, which is slightly alkaline. If the body is in a very acidic state, it will seek balance, and may do so by drawing nutrients from the bones.

*Ama* – Ama refers to toxins that can reside in the body. It is a sticky, toxin substance that is the source of disease.

*Amino Acids* - Amino acids are the building blocks of proteins. In eukaryotes, there are 20 standard amino acids out of which almost all proteins are made.

*Antioxidant* - Antioxidants are substances that can prevent or slow damage to cells caused by free radicals, unstable molecules that the body produces as a reaction to environmental and other pressures. Antioxidants can give up an electron without compromising their inherent structural integrity, thus stopping the oxidative process of free radicals.

*Aparigraha* – This is the fifth of the yamas and refers to restraint from possessiveness and actions motivated by greed.

*ASPCA* - The American Society for the Prevention of Cruelty to Animals (ASPCA) is a non-profit organization dedicated to preventing cruelty to animals.

*Asteya* – This is the third of the yamas and refers to non-stealing behaviours.

*Asthma* - Asthma is a chronic disease involving the airways in the lungs, marked by attacks of spasm in the bronchi of the lungs, causing difficulty in breathing. It is usually connected to allergic reaction or other forms of hypersensitivity.

*Autism* - Autism is a lifelong, non-progressive neurological disorder typically appearing before the age of three years. It is a complex neurobehavioral condition that includes impairments in social interaction and developmental language and communication skills combined with rigid, repetitive behaviours.

*Ayurveda* - The traditional Hindu system of medicine, which is based on the idea of balance in bodily systems and uses diet, herbal treatment, and yogic breathing.

*Benzene* - Benzene is a widely used industrial chemical. Benzene is found in crude oil and is a major part of gasoline. It's used to make plastics, resins, synthetic fibres, rubber lubricants, dyes, detergents, drugs and pesticides. Benzene is a natural by-product of volcanoes and forest fires.

*Beta-Carotene* – Beta-carotene is a vitamin that acts as an antioxidant, protecting cells against oxidation damage. Beta carotene is converted by the body to vitamin A. Food sources of beta carotene include vegetables such as carrots, sweet potatoes, spinach and other leafy green vegetables; and fruit such as cantaloupes and apricots.

*Bile* – Bile is a greenish yellow secretion that is produced in the liver and passed to the gallbladder for concentration, storage, or transport into the first region of the small intestine, the duodenum. Its function is to aid in the digestion of fats in the duodenum.

*Biotin* - Biotin helps release energy from carbohydrates and aids in the metabolism of fats, proteins and carbohydrates from food.

*Body Mass Index (BMI)* - The body mass index (BMI)

is a tool used to assess and monitor changes in body weight. To calculate BMI, divide weight in kilograms (kg) by height in meters squared (m2).

*BPA* – aka bisphenol A, BPA is an industrial chemical that has been used to make certain plastics and resins since the 1960s. BPA is found in polycarbonate plastics and epoxy resins. Polycarbonate plastics are often used in containers that store food and beverages, such as water bottles. BPA can imitate the body's hormones, and it can interfere with the production, secretion, transport, action, function, and elimination of natural hormones. BPA can behave in a similar way to oestrogen and other hormones in the human body.

*Brahmacharya* – This is the fourth of the yamas and refers to restraint from excessive behaviours.
*Calcitonin* – Calcitonin is a hormone secreted by the thyroid that has the effect of lowering blood calcium.

*Calcium* - Calcium is a mineral that is necessary for life. In addition to building bones and keeping them healthy, calcium enables our blood to clot, our muscles to contract, and our heart to beat. About 99% of the calcium in our bodies is in our bones and teeth.

*Calorie* - A calorie is a unit that is used to measure energy. The calorie as it appears on a food package is actually a kilocalorie, or 1,000 calories. A calorie (k-cal) is the amount of energy needed to raise the temperature of one kilogram of water one degree Celsius.

*Candida* – Candida is the name for the genus of yeast that causes fungal infections, known as *candidiasis*. It most commonly occurs as *thrush*, in the mouth and throat, and *yeast infection* in the vagina. Candida yeasts normally reside in the intestinal tract.

*Carbohydrate* - Carbohydrates are the sugars, starches and fibres found in fruits, grains, vegetables and milk products. They are the primary source of energy for the human body.

*Carcinogen* – A carcinogen is any substance that causes cancer in living tissues.

*Cardiovascular Disease* - Cardiovascular disease generally refers to conditions that involve narrowed or blocked blood vessels that can lead to a heart attack, chest pain (angina), or stroke.

*Carotenoids* - Carotenoids are plant pigments responsible for bright red, yellow and orange hues in many fruits and vegetables. They have important antioxidant functions.

*Chloride* - Chloride is one of the most important electrolytes in the blood. It helps keep the amount of fluid inside and outside of your cells in balance. It also helps maintain proper blood volume, blood pressure, and pH of your body fluids.

*Chlorinated Sucrose* – this substance is obtained

through selective substitution of three hydroxyl groups with chlorine atoms, resulting in a substantial increase in sweetness. The result is sucralose, as used in Splenda.

*Chromium* - Chromium is important in the metabolism of fats and carbohydrates. It stimulates fatty acid and cholesterol synthesis, which are important for brain function and other body processes. Chromium also aids in insulin action and glucose metabolism.

*Chyme* – Chyme is the pulpy acidic fluid, which passes from the stomach to the small intestine, consisting of gastric juices and partly digested food.

*Circadian Cycles* - Circadian rhythms are physical, mental, and behavioural changes that follow a daily cycle. They respond primarily to light and darkness in an organism's environment.

*Cobalimin* – *aka vitamin B12*, cobalamin, aids in the building of genetic material, production of normal red blood cells, and maintenance of the nervous system.

*Colitis* – Colitis is a swelling from inflammation of the colon, or large intestine. Food causes can include alcohol, caffeine, dairy products, dried beans, dried fruits, and foods that contain sulphur or sulphate as a preservative.

*Colon* – The colon is part of the large intestine, the

final part of the digestive system. Its function is to reabsorb fluids and process waste products from the body and prepare for its elimination.

*Colostomy* - A colostomy is a surgical procedure that brings one end of the large intestine out through the abdominal wall. During this procedure, one end of the colon is diverted through an incision in the abdominal wall to create a stoma. A stoma is the opening in the skin where a pouch for collecting feces is attached.

*Complex Carbohydrates* - Complex carbohydrates are made up of sugar molecules that are strung together in long, complex chains. Complex carbohydrates are found in foods such as peas, beans, whole grains, and vegetables.

*Copper* - Copper is an essential nutrient for the body. Together with iron, it enables the body to form red blood cells. It helps maintain healthy bones, blood vessels, nerves, and immune function, and it contributes to iron absorption.

*Cortisol* - Cortisol is a steroid hormone that is produced by the adrenal glands. When released into the bloodstream, cortisol can act on many different parts of the body and can help the body respond to stress or danger. It can also increase the body's metabolism of glucose.

*Creatine* - Creatine is a substance that is found naturally in muscle cells. It helps your muscles produce energy during heavy lifting or high-intensity exercise. It is often used by athletes as a "legal steroid" to increase muscle bulk.

*Cryptosporidium* – aka Crypto, is an intestinal infection characterized by diarhhea, caused by a microscopic parasite, Cryptosporidium parvum. The parasite lives in the small intestine of humans and animals, and is passed in their feces. The parasite is protected by an outer shell that allows it to survive outside the body for long periods of time and makes it resistant to chlorine disinfection. Cryptosporidium is one of the most common causes of waterborne disease in the world, including the US. Crypto is transmitted by the fecal-oral route.

*Cytokines* - Cytokines are cell-signalling molecules that aid intercellular communication in immune responses, and stimulate the movement of cells towards sites of inflammation, infection, and trauma.

*Dietary Fibre* - Dietary fibre is a type of carbohydrate that cannot be digested by our bodies' enzymes. It is found in edible plant foods such as cereals, fruits, vegetables, dried peas, nuts, lentils and grains. The main role of dietary fibre is to keep the digestive system healthy by helping to move food through the digestive system.

*Disaccharides* – A disaccharide is the sugar formed when two monosaccharides are joined. These include sucrose, lactose, and maltose.

*Diverticulitis* - Diverticulitis, specifically colonic diverticulitis, is a gastrointestinal disease characterized by inflammation of abnormal pouches, diverticula, which can develop in the wall of the large intestine.

*DNA* - DNA is an acid (deoxyribonucleic acid) in the chromosomes of the cells of living things. DNA determines the particular structure and functions of every cell, and is responsible for characteristics being passed on from parents to their children.

*Dopamine* - Dopamine helps regulate movement, attention, learning, and emotional responses. It enables one to see rewards, and to take action to move toward them. Dopamine is associated with feelings of euphoria, bliss, motivation, and concentration. Dopamine is involved in many pathways in the brain, playing an important role in a range of body systems as well as functions, including movement, sleep, learning, mood, memory, and attention.

*Dosha* - (in Ayurvedic medicine) each of three energies believed to circulate in the body and govern physiological activity, their differing proportions determining individual temperament and physical constitution and (when unbalanced) causing a disposition to particular physical and mental disorders.

*Duodenum* – The duodenum is the first part of the small intestine. It is located between the stomach and the middle part of the small intestine, or jejunum.

*E. coli* – This bacterium commonly found in the intestines of humans and other animals, some strains of which can cause severe food poisoning. E. coli infection can happen by coming into contact with the feces, or stool, of humans or animals. This can occur when drinking water or eating food that has been contaminated by feces. E. coli can get into meat during processing.

*Eight Limbs of Yoga* - Patanjali's Eight Limbs of Yoga offers guidelines for a meaningful and purposeful life. This includes Yama (moral restraints), Niyama (personal observances), Asana (physical postures), Pranayama (breath), Pratyahara (withdrawal of the senses), Dharana (concentration), Dhyana (meditation), and Samadhi (complete integration).

*Electrolyte* – Electrolytes are minerals in your body that have an electric charge. These include sodium, potassium, chloride, calcium, magnesium, and phosphate. They are in your blood, urine, tissues, and other body fluids. Electrolytes help to balance the amount of water in your body, as well as the body's acid/base (pH) level.

*Endocrine Gland* - Endocrine glands are glands of the endocrine system that secrete their products, hormones, directly into the blood rather than through a duct. The major glands of the endocrine system include the pineal gland, pituitary gland, pancreas, ovaries, testes, thyroid gland, para-thyroid gland, hypothalamus and adrenal glands.

*Endocrine System* - The endocrine system is a chemical messenger system consisting of hormones, the group of glands of an organism that secrete those hormones directly into the circulatory system to regulate the function of distant target organs, and the feedback loops which modulate hormone release so that homeostasis is maintained.

*Enteroendocrine Cells* - Enteroendocrine cells are cells found in the wall of the gut that secrete hormones that regulate numerous processes in the body, including controlling glucose levels, food intake, and stomach emptying.

*Enzyme* - Enzymes are biological molecules (typically proteins) that significantly speed up the rate of virtually all of the chemical reactions that take place within cells. They are vital for life and serve a wide range of important functions in the body, such as aiding in digestion and metabolism.

*Epilepsy* - Epilepsy is a common condition that affects the brain and causes frequent seizures. Seizures are bursts of electrical activity in the brain that temporarily affect how it works. They can cause a wide range of symptoms. Epilepsy can start at any age, but usually starts either in childhood or in people over 60.

*Essential Amino Acids* - Essential Amino Acids are not

made by the body, and must be acquired from food sources.

*Ethics* – Ethics refers to rules of behaviour based on ideas about what is morally good and bad.

*Exocrine Gland* - Exocrine glands are glands that produce and secrete substances onto an epithelial surface by way of a duct, including sweat, salivary, and mammary glands.

*Factory Farming* – This is animal agriculture, involving a large industrialized farm, especially one on which large numbers of livestock are raised inside in conditions intended to maximize production at minimal cost.

*Fat-soluble vitamins* – Fat-soluble vitamins dissolve in fat before they are absorbed in the bloodstream to carry out their functions. They are vitamins A, D, E, and K.

*Fecal Contamination* - The presence of fecal coliform in aquatic environments may indicate that the water has been contaminated with the fecal material of humans or other animals. Fecal coliform bacteria can enter rivers through direct discharge of waste from mammals and birds, from agricultural and storm runoff, and from human sewage.

*Fight or Flight* - The *fight or flight response* (also called hyper-arousal, or the acute stress response) is a physiological reaction that occurs in response to a perceived harmful event, attack, or threat to survival.

*Fluoride* - Fluoride occurs naturally in the body as calcium fluoride. Calcium fluoride is mostly found in the bones and teeth. Excess fluoride in the body can be disruptive to thyroid function.

*Folate* – aka vitamin B9 or folic acid, folate aids in protein metabolism, promoting red blood cell formation, and lowering the risk for neural tube birth defects. Folate may also play a role in controlling homocysteine levels, thus reducing the risk for coronary heart disease.

*Food and Drug Administration (FDA)* - The FDA is an agency within the U.S. Department of Health and Human Services (HHS) that oversees the manufacturing and distribution of food, pharmaceuticals, medical devices, tobacco and other consumer products, and veterinary medicine.

*Free Radical* - Free radicals are molecules with unpaired electrons. Electrons like to be in pairs, so these atoms, called free radicals, scavenge the body to seek out other electrons so they can become a pair. Free radicals can cause damage to parts of cells such as proteins, DNA, and cell membranes by stealing their electrons through a process called oxidation.

*Fructose* - Fructose is a monosaccharide (simple

sugar), which occurs naturally in fruit, vegetables, and honey.

*Gallbladder* – The gallbladder is a small hollow organ where bile is stored and concentrated before it is released into the small intestine.

*Ghrelin* - Ghrelin is a hormone that is produced and released mainly by the stomach with small amounts also released by the small intestine, pancreas and brain. Ghrelin has numerous functions. It is termed the 'hunger hormone' because it stimulates appetite, increases food intake and promotes fat storage.

*Glucagon* - Glucagon is a hormone produced by the pancreas that causes the liver to release glucose into the blood. It is used to quickly increase blood sugar levels.

*Glucocorticoids* – A glucocorticoid is any steroid hormone that is produced by the adrenal gland and is known particularly for its anti-inflammatory and immunosuppressive actions.

*Glucose* – Glucose is a monosaccharide (simple sugar), which is an important energy source in living organisms and is a component of many carbohydrates.

*Gluten* - Gluten is a general name for the proteins found in wheat, rye, and barley. Gluten helps foods maintain their shape, acting as the glue that holds food together. In people with celiac disease, gluten triggers an immune response that damages the lining of the small intestine. This can interfere with the absorption of nutrients from food. Gluten sensitivity is a more common ailment, and difficult to diagnose. It can lead to digestive discomfort, and trigger an immune response upon consumption of products containing gluten.

*Glycogen* - Glycogen is a form of glucose that is stored, mainly in the liver and the muscles, in for future use. When energy is needed, glycogen is quickly mobilized to deliver the fuel that the body needs.

*Gonads* - Gonads are the male and female primary reproductive organs. The male gonads are the testes and the female gonads are the ovaries.

*Growth Hormones (HGH)* - HGH, produced by the pituitary gland, spurs growth in children and adolescents. It also helps to regulate body composition, body fluids, muscle and bone growth, sugar and fat metabolism, and possibly heart function.

*Gunas* - A guna is an attribute of nature, according to Hindu philosophy. In Hinduism, there are three gunas that have always existed in the world in both all living and non-living things.

*Heterocyclic Amines* – aka HCA, heterocyclic amines are carcinogens. This term refers to a chemical that is formed when meat, poultry, or fish is cooked at high temperatures, including frying, broiling, or barbecuing.

*High Fructose Corn Syrup (HFCS)* – HFCS is a sweetener made from cornflour, some of whose glucose has been converted to fructose. It is used in commercially produced foods and soft drinks as a cheaper alternative to sucrose. It is metabolized to fat in the body far more rapidly than any other sugar, and, because most fructose is consumed in liquid form, its negative metabolic effects are significantly magnified. This processed sweetener is found in thousands of packaged and processed foods and beverages.

*Holistic* – A philosophy characterized by the belief that the parts of something are intimately interconnected and explicable only by reference to the whole; a medical practice characterized by the treatment of the whole person, taking into account mental and social factors, rather than just the symptoms of a disease.

*Homeostasis* – Homeostasis is the ability or tendency of a living organism, cell, or group to keep the conditions inside it the same despite any changes in the conditions around it. It is the maintenance of a state of internal balance.

*Hormone* - Hormones are special chemical messengers in the body that are created in the endocrine glands. These messengers control most major bodily functions, from simple basic needs like hunger to complex systems like reproduction, and even the emotions and mood.

*Hydrogenation* - Hydrogenation is a process in which a liquid unsaturated fat is turned into a solid fat by adding hydrogen. Food companies began using hydrogenated oil to help increase shelf life and save costs. During this manufactured, partially hydrogenated processing, a type of fat called trans fat is made.

*Hypothalamus* – The hypothalamus coordinates both the autonomic nervous system and the activity of the pituitary, controlling body temperature, thirst, hunger, and other homeostatic systems, and is involved in sleep and emotional activity.

*Ileum* – The ileum is part of the small intestine beyond the jejunum and before the large intestine (colon). It accounts for approximately three fifths of the length of the small intestine, and is the primary site of the absorption of vitamin B12 and bile salts.

*Ileostomy* - An ileostomy is an opening in the belly (abdominal wall) that's made during surgery. The end of the ileum (the lowest part of the small intestine) is brought through this opening to form a stoma, usually on the lower right side of the abdomen.

*Inflammation* - Inflammation is part of the complex biological response of body tissues to harmful stimuli, such as pathogens, damaged cells, or irritants, and is a protective response involving immune cells, blood vessels, and molecular mediators.

*Insoluble Fibre* - Insoluble fibre does not absorb or dissolve in water. It passes through the digestive system in close to its original form.
It adds bulk to the stool, and appears to help food pass more quickly through the stomach and intestines.

*Insulin* - Insulin is a hormone made by the pancreas that allows the body to use sugar (glucose) from carbohydrates for energy, or to store glucose for future use. Insulin helps to keep blood sugar levels from getting too high.

*Insulin-like Growth Factor 1 (IGF-1)* - A protein made by the body that stimulates the growth of many types of cells. High levels of IGF-1 may increase the risk of several types of cancer. Insulin-like growth factor is a type of cytokine.

*Insulin Resistance* – This condition is an impaired response of the body to the effects of insulin, resulting in elevated levels of glucose in the blood, which is a key component of Type-2 diabetes and metabolic syndrome.
Elevated free fatty acid levels (due to obesity or to high-fat nutritional habits) cause insulin resistance in skeletal muscle and the liver, which contributes to the development of Type-2 diabetes, and produces low-grade inflammation, which contributes to the development of atherosclerotic vascular diseases.

*Iodine* - The body needs iodine to make thyroid hormones. These hormones control the body's metabolism and many other important functions.

*Iron* - Iron is an essential element for blood production. About 70 percent of your body's iron is found in the red blood cells of your blood called hemoglobin and in muscle cells called myoglobin. Hemoglobin is essential for transferring oxygen in your blood from the lungs to the tissues.

*Irritable Bowel Syndrome (IBS)* - Irritable bowel syndrome (IBS) is a group of symptoms that occur together, including repeated pain in the abdomen and changes in bowel movements, which may be diarrhea, constipation, or both. With IBS, these symptoms can exist without any visible signs of damage or disease in your digestive tract.

*Jejunum* – The jejunum is the middle part of the small intestine. It is between the duodenum (first part of the small intestine) and the ileum (last part of the small intestine). The jejunum helps to further digest food coming from the stomach. It absorbs nutrients (vitamins, minerals, carbohydrates, fats, proteins) and water from food.

*Kapha* – One of the doshas. Kapha is the watery element, and is characterized by heaviness, tenderness, softness, and is the carrier of nutrients. It is the nourishing element of the body.

*Kidneys* - The kidneys are a pair of organs that are

found on either side of the spine, just below the rib cage in the back. Kidneys filter waste materials out of the blood and pass them out of the body as urine. They regulate blood pressure and the levels of water, salts, and minerals in the body.

*Kidney Stones* - Kidney stones have many causes and can affect any part of your urinary tract, from your kidneys to your bladder. Stones can form when the urine becomes concentrated, allowing minerals to crystallize and stick together.

*Lactose* – Lactose is a sugar present in milk. It is a disaccharide containing glucose and galactose units.

*Lactose Intolerance* - Lactose intolerance is the inability to digest lactose, a component of milk and some other dairy products. The basis for lactose intolerance is the lack of an enzyme called lactase in the small intestine. The most common symptoms of lactose intolerance are diarrhea, bloating, and gas.

*Larynx* – The larynx houses vocal folds, and manipulates pitch and volume of the voice. It is known as the *voice box.*

*Leaky Gut* - Leaky gut, also known as increased intestinal permeability, is a condition in which the lining of the small intestine becomes damaged, causing undigested food particles, toxic waste products and bacteria to "leak" through the intestines and flood the blood stream. Intestinal permeability can be responsible for chronic inflammation. The foreign substances that get into the blood are recognised as pathogens and handled accordingly by the immune system. This on-going situation can result in chronic fatigue, and a continued immune response, which may contribute to various diseases.

*Leptin* - A hormone produced mainly by fat cells in the adipose tissue that is involved in the regulation of body fat. Leptin interacts with areas of the brain that control hunger and behaviour and signals that the body has had enough to eat.

*Leukemia* – Leukemia is a malignant progressive disease in which the bone marrow and other blood-forming organs produce increased numbers of immature or abnormal leucocytes.

*Liver* – The liver is the largest solid organ in the body, and is situated in the upper part of the abdomen on the right side. The liver has a multitude of important and complex functions: to manufacture proteins, including albumin (to help maintain the volume of blood) and blood clotting factors; to synthesize, store, and process fats, including fatty acids (used for energy) and cholesterol; to metabolize and store carbohydrates as glycogen (used as the source for the sugar in blood); to form and secrete bile that contains bile acids, which aid in the intestinal absorption of fats and the fat-soluble vitamins A, D, E, and K; to eliminate, by metabolizing or secreting, the potentially harmful biochemical products produced by the body, such as bilirubin, from the breakdown of old red blood cells and ammonia from the breakdown of proteins; and to detoxify, by metabolizing and/or secreting, drugs, alcohol, and environmental toxins.

*Lutein* – Lutein is a yellow carotenoid pigment, and a potent antioxidant.

*Lycopene* - Lycopene is a powerful antioxidant with many health benefits, including sun protection, improved heart health, and a lower risk of certain types of cancer.

*Lymphatic System* - The lymphatic system is part of the immune system. It is a network of tissues and organs that help rid the body of toxins, waste, and other unwanted materials. The primary function of the lymphatic system is to transport lymph, a fluid containing infection-fighting white blood cells, throughout the body.

*Lymphoma* - Lymphoma is cancer that begins in infection-fighting cells of the immune system, called lymphocytes. IT can affect some or all of the organs of the lymphatic system.

*Macronutrients* – Macronutrients are types of food that are required in large amounts in nutritional intake. These include carbohydrates, fats, and proteins.

*Maltodextrin* - Maltodextrin is a white, starchy powder that food manufacturers add into many food items to improve their flavour, thickness, or shelf life. It originates from corn, rice, potato starch, or wheat. It is a highly processed food additive.

*Maltose* - a sugar produced by the breakdown of starch, by enzymes found in malt and saliva. It is a disaccharide consisting of two linked glucose units.

*Magnesium* – Magnesium is a mineral involved in many processes in the body including nerve signalling, the building of healthy bones, and normal muscle contraction. About 350 enzymes are known to depend on magnesium.

*Major Minerals* – The major minerals are calcium, sodium, potassium, magnesium, phosphorus, chloride, and sulfur.

*Manganese* - It aids in the formation of connective tissue, bones, blood-clotting factors, and sex hormones and plays a role in fat and carbohydrate metabolism, calcium absorption, and blood sugar regulation. Manganese is also necessary for normal brain and nerve function.

*Melatonin* - Melatonin plays an important role in the regulation of sleep cycles (circadian rhythm). Its production is influenced by the detection of light and dark by the retina of the eye.

*Methionine* - One of the major roles of methionine in the body is that it can be used to produce other important molecules. It is involved in the production of cysteine, the other sulphur containing amino acids used to build proteins in the body

*Mercury – This heavy metal is a by-product of fossil fuel combustion.*

*Methanol* – This substance is a neurotoxin, which breaks down into formaldehyde when heated over 30 degrees Celcius (86 Farenheit).

*Methylmercury* – Methylmercury refers to compounds that often occur as pollutants, which accumulate in living organisms (such as fish) especially in higher levels of a food chain.

*Microbiome* – Microbiome is a community of micro-organisms, including bacteria, fungi, and viruses, which inhabit and live in a particular environment in the human body. The human microbiome, located in the colon, helps with food digestion, produces certain vitamins, regulates our immune systems, and fights against disease-causing bacteria.

*Micronutrients* – Micronutrients are one of the major groups of nutrients that are required by the body. These vitamins and minerals are required in very small amounts. Vitamins are necessary for energy production, immune function, blood clotting and other functions. Minerals play an important role in growth, bone health, fluid balance and several other processes.

*Microplastics* – These are extremely small pieces of plastic debris in the environment, resulting from the disposal and breakdown of consumer products and industrial waste.

*Milk Allergy* - Milk allergy is an adverse immune reaction to one or more proteins in cow's milk. When allergy symptoms occur, they can occur rapidly or have a gradual onset. It is due to the absence of lactase (the enzyme required to break down the lactose present in animal milk), the levels of which naturally decline after childhood.

*Mineral* - A mineral is a chemical element required as an essential nutrient by organisms to perform functions necessary for life. The five major minerals in the human body are calcium, phosphorus, potassium, sodium, and magnesium.

*Mineralcorticoids* - Mineralcorticoids are a corticosteroid that primarily affects the electrolyte and fluid balance in the body.

*Mitochondria* - Mitochondria are known as the powerhouses of the cell. They are organelles that act like a digestive system, which takes in nutrients, breaks them down, and creates energy rich molecules for the cell.

*Molybdenum* - Molybdenum is an essential nutrient. Its main function is in removing toxins particularly from the metabolism of sulfur containing amino acids.

*Monosaccharides* - A monosaccharide is the most basic form of carbohydrates. These include glucose, dextrose, fructose, and galactose.

*Monounsaturated Fat* - Monounsaturated fats are found in plant foods, such as avocados, nuts, and vegetable oils. These foods have multiple health benefits; however, they must be consumed in moderation due to their high fat content.

*Neurotoxin* – A neurotoxin is a poisonous substance that disrupts and alters the structure or function of the nervous systems. Long-term effects can include widespread central nervous system damage, including intellectual disability, persistent memory impairments, epilepsy, and dementia. More than 1,000 chemicals are known to have neurotoxic effects in animals.

*Niacin* – *aka vitamin B3*, niacin is involved in energy production, normal enzyme function, digestion, promoting normal appetite, healthy skin, and nerves.

*Niyamas* – This is the second of the Eight Limbs of Yoga and refers to the restraints in attitudes toward the self.

*Noradrenalin* – Noradrenalin is a hormone, which is released by the adrenal medulla and by the sympathetic nerves and functions as a neurotransmitter. It is also used as a drug to raise blood pressure. The sympathetic nervous system triggers a response that is commonly referred to as our 'fight or flight response.'

*Obesity* - Obesity is defined as abnormal or excessive fat accumulation that presents a risk to health. Generally thought to be in excess of 20% over ideal body weight.

*Oesophagus* - The oesophagus is a long, muscular tube that connects your mouth to your stomach. It's around 25cm (10in) long in adults.

*Oestrogen* - any of a group of steroid hormones, which promote the development and maintenance of female characteristics of the body.

*Omega 3* – Omega 3 fatty acids, which can be found in foods, act to reduce levels of LDL cholesterol (the bad kind). These are known to improve risk factors for heart disease, and can fight depression and anxiety.

*Omega 6* - Omega-6 fatty acids are used for reducing the risk of heart disease, lowering total cholesterol levels, lowering LDL cholesterol levels, raising HDL cholesterol levels, and reducing cancer risk. Too much omega 6 can raise blood pressure, lead to blood clots that can cause heart attack and stroke, and cause the body to retain water.

*Opioid Peptides* - Opioid peptides bind to opioid receptors in the brain. Opiates and opioids mimic the effect of these peptides. Opiates include codeine, morphine, heroin, opium, Oxycodone, and Percocet).

*Ovaries* - The ovaries are an important part of the female reproductive system. Their job is twofold. They produce the hormones, including oestrogen, that trigger menstruation. They also release at least one egg each month for possible fertilization.

*Oxidative Stress* - Oxidative stress is an imbalance between free radicals and antioxidants in your body. Oxidative stress can cause damage to DNA strands, and can lead to many ailments, including neurodegenerative diseases such as Parkinson's disease and Alzheimer's disease, gene mutations and cancers, chronic fatigue syndrome, heart and blood vessel disorders, atherosclerosis, heart failure, heart attack, and inflammatory diseases.

*Oxytocin* - Oxytocin, otherwise known as the love hormone, is released by the pituitary gland and is responsible for human behaviours associated with relationships and bonding. It is responsible for producing contractions in labour and controlling bleeding.

*Palmitate* – Palmitate is the major fatty acid found in palm oil. It can initiate oxidative stress in adipose tissue.

*Pancreas* - The pancreas is an organ located in the abdomen. It plays an essential role in converting food into fuel for the body's cells. The pancreas has two main functions: an exocrine function that helps in digestion and an endocrine function that regulates blood sugar.

*Pantothenic Acid* – aka vitamin B5, Pantothenic Acid is involved in energy production, and aids in the formation of hormones and the metabolism of fats, proteins, and carbohydrates from food.

*Parathyroid Glands* - The parathyroid glands are four tiny glands, located in the neck, that help to control the body's calcium levels.

*Parathyroid hormone (PTH)* - When the calcium in our blood goes too low, the parathyroid glands make more PTH. Increased PTH causes the bones to release their calcium into the blood.

*Pathogen* – A pathogen is a bacterium, virus, or other microorganism that can cause disease.

*Peristalsis* - Peristalsis is a series of wave-like muscle contractions that moves food to different processing stations in the digestive tract.

*Pineal Gland* - The pineal gland produces melatonin, a serotonin-derived hormone, which modulates sleep patterns in both circadian and seasonal cycles. French philosopher, Réné Descartes, called it "the seat of the soul."

*Pituitary Gland* – The pituitary is the major endocrine

gland, a pea-sized body that is attached to the base of the brain. It is important in controlling growth and development and the influences the functioning of the other endocrine glands.

*pH level* - pH is a measurement of how acidic or alkaline (basic) a substance is. The scale runs from 0 to 14. A pH of less than 7 is considered acidic, and a pH of more than 7 is basic. Overly acidic levels in the body's pH can create a physically stressful environment, which requires using calcium resources to re-establish a healthy pH level. An overly alkaline state is equally unfavourable foe the human body.

*Phosphorus* - Phosphorus is a mineral that makes up 1% of a person's total body weight. It is the second most abundant mineral in the body. It is present in every cell of the body. Most of the phosphorus in the body is found in the bones and teeth.

*Phytic Acid* – Phytic acid is a unique natural substance found in plant seeds. High concentrations exist in the bran part of wheat.
Phytic acid impairs the absorption of iron, zinc, and calcium and may promote mineral deficiencies. Soaking grains, rice, and beans before preparation and consumption can reduce the levels of phytic acid.

*Phytonutrient*  -  Phytonutrients,  also called phytochemicals, are chemicals produced by plants. Phytonutrients can also provide significant benefits for humans who eat plant foods. Phytonu-

trient-rich foods include colourful fruits and vegetables, legumes, nuts, tea, whole grains and many
spices.

*Pitta* – One of the doshas. Pitta governs metabolism
and transformation in the body. Its chief quality is
heat. It is the energy principle, which uses bile to direct digestion and enhance metabolism.

*Polysaccharides* - a carbohydrate (starch, cellulose, or
glycogen) whose molecules consist of a number of
sugar molecules bonded together. A polysaccharide
is a large molecule consisting of many smaller monosaccharides.

*Polyunsaturated Fat* - Polyunsaturated fats can help reduce LDL cholesterol levels, thus lowering the risk
of heart disease and stroke. Oils rich in polyunsaturated fats also provide essential fats that the body requires, but cannot produce itself – such as omega-6
and omega-3 fatty acids.

*Potassium* - Potassium is an important mineral that
functions as an electrolyte. It helps regulate fluid balance, nerve signals and muscle contractions.

*Prana* – Prana can refer to energy, life, or breath. It is
the universal sea of energy that infuses and vitalizes
all matter.

*Processed Food* - A processed food is a food item that
has had a series of mechanical or chemical oper-

ations performed on it to change or preserve it.

*Progesterone* - Progesterone is one of the progesterone steroid hormones. It is secreted by the corpus luteum, a temporary endocrine gland that the female body produces after ovulation during the second half of the menstrual cycle. Progesterone prepares the body for pregnancy.

*Protein* - Protein is a nutrient found in food that is made up of many amino acids joined together, is a necessary part of the diet, and is essential for normal cell structure and function.

*Pyridoxine* – *aka vitamin B6*, pyridoxal or pyridoxamine, this vitamin compound aids in protein metabolism and red blood cell formation. It is also involved in the body's production of chemicals such as insulin and haemoglobin.

*Rajas* – Rajas is one of the three gunas, and translates as *passion*.
*Recommended Daily Amount (RDA)* - Recommended Dietary Allowance is the average daily level of intake sufficient to meet the nutrient requirements of nearly all (97%-98%) healthy people.

*Resveratrol* - A polyphenol compound found in certain plants that has antioxidant properties, and has been investigated for possible anti-carcinogenic effects.

*Rheumatoid Arthritis* – Rheumatoid arthritis is an

autoimmune condition, which means that it is caused by the immune system attacking body tissue. It causes inflammation in the joints, and can result in painful deformity and immobility, especially in the fingers, wrists, feet, and ankles.

*Riboflavin – aka vitamin B2*, riboflavin facilitates the release of energy from foods, promotes good vision, and maintains healthy skin. It also helps to convert the amino acid tryptophan (which makes up protein) into niacin.

*Salivary Response* – Salivary response is an autonomic response of the salivary glands to produce saliva. This is the first step of the digestive process, and can be triggered by the thoughts, smell, sight, or taste of food.

*Salmonella* - Salmonella refers to a group of bacteria that cause Salmonella infection in the intestinal tract. Salmonella poisoning is often linked to contaminated water or foods, especially meat, poultry, and eggs.

*Samprapti* – The Sanskrit word from *samyak* "proper" and *prapti* "to get." Samprapti is to get the proper knowledge about the pathway of disease manifestation.

*Satiety* – Satiety is the state of being completely satisfied, especially with food or pleasure, so that you could not have any more.

*Sattva* - Sattva is one of the three gunas. Sattva denotes having the natural quality of purity and goodness.

*Saturated Fat* - Like other fats, saturated fat contains nine calories per gram. Saturated fats contain a high proportion of saturated fatty acids, which contain no double bonds. Saturated fats are solid at room temperature, and include those fats found in butter, cheese, red meat and other animal-based foods. These fats are known to raise LDL cholesterol levels and a higher risk for heart disease.

*Satya* – This is the second of the yamas and refers to actions of truthfulness.

*Schizophrenia* – Schizophrenia is a long-term mental disorder of a type involving a breakdown in the relation between thought, emotion, and behaviour, leading to faulty perception, inappropriate actions and feelings, withdrawal from reality and personal relationships into fantasy and delusion, and a sense of mental fragmentation.

*Selenium* - Selenium helps your body make special proteins, called antioxidant enzymes. These play a role in preventing cell damage.

*Small Intestine* - The small intestine is the part of the

gastrointestinal tract between the stomach and the large intestine, and is where most of the end absorption of food takes place. The small intestine has three distinct regions – the duodenum, jejunum, and ileum.

*Sodium* - Sodium is an essential electrolyte that helps maintain the balance of water in and around your cells. It's important for proper muscle and nerve function. It also helps maintain stable blood pressure levels.

*Soluble Fibre* - Soluble fibre attracts water and turns to gel during digestion. This slows digestion, which promotes nutrient absorption. Soluble fibre is found in oat bran, barley, nuts, seeds, beans, lentils, peas, and some fruits and vegetables.

*Stomach* - The stomach is a muscular organ located on the left side of the upper abdomen. The stomach receives food from the oesophagus. It secretes acid and enzymes that digest food. Ridges of muscle tissue called rugae line the stomach. The stomach muscles contract periodically, churning food to enhance digestion.

*Sucrose* - Sucrose is a disaccharide of glucose and fructose obtained from sugar cane and sugar beet, used as a sweetener. Sucrose is common table sugar.

*Sulfur* - Sulfur is crucial to many of the most important functions in your body, including joint health, insulin function and energy production. IT is the third most abundant mineral in the body behind calcium and phosphorus.

*Sulphuric Acid* – aka Vitriol, sulphuric acid widely used in fertilisers, as well as in the production of hydrochloric acid, nitric acid, sulfate salts, synthetic detergents, dyes and pigments, explosives, and drugs.

*Superfood* – This term refers to a nutrient-rich food considered to be especially beneficial for health and wellbeing.

*Sustainability* – Sustainability is the quality of being able to continue over a period of time, and also refers to the quality of causing little or no damage to the environment.

*Tamas* – Tamas is one of the three gunas. It translates as *darkness, illusion,* and *ignorance*

*Telomere* - Telomeres function to protect the ends of chromosomes from sticking to each other. They also protect genetic information during cell division because a short piece of each chromosome is lost every time DNA is replicated.

*Testes* - The testes (or testicles) are a pair of sperm-producing organs that maintain the health of the male reproductive system.

*Testosterone* - Testosterone is the key male sex hormone that regulates fertility, muscle mass, fat distribution, and red blood cell production.

*T-lymphocytes* - T lymphocytes are part of the immune system and develop from stem cells in the bone marrow. They help protect the body from infection and may help fight cancer. Also known as T cells.

*Thiamin – aka vitamin B1*, thiamin helps to release energy from foods, promotes normal appetite, and is important in maintaining proper nervous system function.

*Thymosin* – Thymosin is one of several polypeptide hormones secreted by the thymus that control the maturation of T cells.

*Thymus* – The thymus is an organ that is located in the upper chest behind the breastbone and in front of the lower neck in which the immune cells called T lymphocytes mature and multiply in early life. The thymus begins to shrink after puberty.

*Thyroid Gland* - The thyroid gland produces hormones that regulate the body's metabolic rate as well as heart and digestive function, muscle control, brain development, mood and bone maintenance. Its correct functioning depends on having a good supply of iodine from the diet. The thyroid gland also plays a role in the absorption of calcium.

*Thyroxin* - Thyroxine is a hormone that the thyroid gland secretes into the bloodstream. Thyroxine plays a crucial role in heart and digestive function, growth and metabolism, brain development, bone health, and muscle control. It affects almost all of the body's systems.

*Trace Minerals* - Trace minerals are important in body functions, though are needed in much smaller amounts. Trace minerals include iron, chromium, copper, zinc, iodine, manganese, and selenium.

*Type-2 Diabetes* – aka diabetes mellitus type 2, is a long-term metabolic disorder that is characterised by high blood sugar, insulin resistance, and resulting lack of insulin effectiveness. It primarily occurs as a result of obesity and lack of exercise.

*U.S. Department of Agriculture (USDA)* - The United States Department of Agriculture (USDA) is the department of the United States government that manages various programs related to food, agriculture, natural resources, rural development and nutrition. Technically, the USDA is responsible for the safety of meat, poultry and egg products, while the FDA regulates all other foods.

*Vata* – One of the doshas. Vata governs all movement in the mind and body. It controls blood flow, elimination of wastes, breathing and the movement of thoughts across the mind. Since Pitta and Kapha cannot move without it, Vata is considered the leader of the three Ayurvedic Principles in the body.

*Vayus* - Through their exploration of the body and

breath, the ancient yogis discovered that prana (life force energy) could be further subdivided into energetic components they called Vayus (winds).

*Vitamin* – Vitamins are a group of substances that are found naturally in many foods, are necessary in small quantities for good health and normal development and functioning, and are designated by a capital letter and sometimes a number, vitamin B6 vitamin C.

*Vitamin A* - Vitamin A, also called retinol, has many functions in the body. In addition to helping the eyes adjust to light changes, vitamin A plays an important role in bone growth, tooth development, reproduction, cell division, gene expression, and regulation of the immune system. The skin, eyes, and mucous membranes depend on vitamin A to remain moist. Vitamin A is also an important antioxidant that may play a role in the prevention of certain cancers.

*Vitamin B1* – aka thiamin, vitamin B1 helps to release energy from foods, promotes normal appetite, and is important in maintaining proper nervous system function.

*Vitamin B2* – aka riboflavin, vitamin B2 facilitates the release of energy from foods, promotes good vision, and maintains healthy skin. It also helps to convert the amino acid tryptophan (which makes up protein) into niacin.

*Vitamin B3* – aka niacin, vitamin B3 is involved in energy production, normal enzyme function, digestion, promoting normal appetite, healthy skin, and nerves.

*Vitamin B5* – aka pantothenic acid, this vitamin is involved in energy production, and aids in the formation of hormones and the metabolism of fats, proteins, and carbohydrates from food.

*Vitamin B6* - aka pyridoxine, pyridoxal or pyridoxamine, this vitamin compound aids in protein metabolism and red blood cell formation. It is also involved in the body's production of chemicals such as insulin and haemoglobin.

*Vitamin B9* – aka folate or folic acid, this vitamin compound aids in protein metabolism, promoting red blood cell formation, and lowering the risk for neural tube birth defects. Vitamin B9 may also play a role in controlling homocysteine levels, thus reducing the risk for coronary heart disease.

*Vitamin B12* – aka cobalamin, vitamin B12 aids in the building of genetic material, production of normal red blood cells, and maintenance of the nervous system.

*Vitamin C* - The body needs vitamin C, also known as ascorbic acid or ascorbate, to remain in proper working condition. Vitamin C benefits the body by holding cells together through collagen synthesis; collagen is a connective tissue that holds muscles, bones, and other tissues together. Vitamin C also aids in wound healing, bone and tooth formation, strengthening blood vessel walls, improving immune system function, increasing absorption and utilization of iron, and acting as an antioxidant. Vitamin C works with vitamin E as an antioxidant, and plays a crucial role in neutralizing free radicals throughout the body. *(Advanced Nutrition: Macronutrients, Micronutrients, and Metabolism (2009). CRC Press, Taylor & Francis Group).*

*Vitamin D* - Vitamin D plays a critical role in the body's use of calcium and phosphorous. It works by increasing the amount of calcium absorbed from the small intestine, helping to form and maintain bones. Vitamin D benefits the body by playing a role in immunity and controlling cell growth.

*Vitamin E* - Vitamin E benefits the body by acting as an antioxidant, and protecting vitamins A and C, red blood cells, and essential fatty acids from destruction.

*Vitamin K* - Vitamin K is naturally produced by the bacteria in the intestines, and plays an essential role in normal blood clotting, promoting bone health, and helping to produce proteins for blood, bones, and kidneys.

*Water-soluble Vitamins* - Water-soluble vitamins can dissolve in water, and are carried to the body's tissues but are not stored in the body. They include vitamin C and the B-complex vitamins.

*Yoga Sutras of Patanjali* - The Yoga *Sutras* are a collection of texts written by the sage, Patanjali, around 400 C.E. The collection contains what is thought to be much of the basis of classical yoga philosophy.

*Yamas* – This is first of the Eight Limbs of Yoga, and refers to restraints in behaviours toward our environment.

*Zinc* - Zinc is found in cells throughout the body. It is needed in order for the immune system to properly work. It plays a role in cell division, cell growth, wound healing, and the breakdown of carbohydrates. Zinc is also needed for the senses of smell and taste.

# ACKNOWLEDGEMENTS

This book would not exist without Candace Stime. Her perpetual inspiration and unwavering support has allowed me to overcome the doubts that can accompany the undertaking of a project like the writing of this book. Her belief, encouragement, and love are humbling. Thank you for always confirming the choice to take risks, and for taking them with me.

Every creative undertaking in my life has been accompanied by the encouragements of my aunt and uncle, Lorna and Marque Neal. From my earliest childhood endeavors to the pursuit of goals throughout my adult life, they were honest, loving, and encouraging. While their passing has left an absence in my worldly consciousness, the memory of their lives remains a thriving source of inspiration.

I would like to thank Glenn Street for the continuous although sometimes distant dialog that we have maintained over the years. The on-going discussion that we have kept going has always been thought provoking and nourishing.

I would also like to express my gratitude to Jennifer Gooch Hummer for her professional and creative contributions to this project. Her experience has been invaluable and has allowed me to get over some of the final hurdles of publishing this book.

www.ingramcontent.com/pod-product-compliance
Lightning Source LLC
Chambersburg PA
CBHW051344280526
45784CB00007B/2808